Grief and Prolonged Grief Disorder

Grief and Prolonged Grief Disorder

Charles F. Reynolds, III, M.D.
Stephen J. Cozza, M.D.
Paul K. Maciejewski, Ph.D.
Holly G. Prigerson, Ph.D.
M. Katherine Shear, M.D.
Naomi M. Simon, M.D., M.Sc.
Sidney Zisook, M.D.

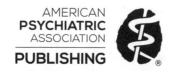

AMERICAN
PSYCHIATRIC
ASSOCIATION
PUBLISHING®

If you wish to buy 50 or more copies of the same title, please go to www.appi.org/special-discounts for more information.

Copyright © 2023 American Psychiatric Association Publishing

ALL RIGHTS RESERVED

First Edition

Manufactured in the United States of America on acid-free paper
27 26 25 24 23   5 4 3 2 1

American Psychiatric Association Publishing
800 Maine Avenue SW, Suite 900
Washington, DC 20024-2812
www.appi.org

Library of Congress Cataloging-in-Publication Data
Names: Reynolds, Charles F., III, 1947- editor. | American Psychiatric Association, issuing body.
Title: Grief and prolonged grief disorder / [edited by] Charles F. Reynolds, III, Stephen J. Cozza, Paul K. Maciejewski, Holly G. Prigerson, Katherine Shear, Naomi Simon, Sidney Zisook.
Description: First edition. | Washington, D.C. : American Psychiatric Association Publishing, [2024] | Includes bibliographical references and index.
Identifiers: LCCN 2023015041 (print) | LCCN 2023015042 (ebook) | ISBN 9781615374632 (paperback) | ISBN 9781615374649 (ebook)
Subjects: MESH: Prolonged Grief Disorder | Grief
Classification: LCC BF575.G7 (print) | LCC BF575.G7 (ebook) | NLM WM 140 | DDC 155.9/37--dc23/eng/20230516
LC record available at https://lccn.loc.gov/2023015041
LC ebook record available at https://lccn.loc.gov/2023015042

British Library Cataloguing in Publication Data
A CIP record is available from the British Library.

Contents

Charles F. Reynolds, III, M.D.
Stephen J. Cozza, M.D.
Paul K. Maciejewski, Ph.D.
Holly G. Prigerson, Ph.D.
M. Katherine Shear, M.D.
Naomi M. Simon, M.D.
Sidney Zisook, M.D.
Natalia A. Skritskaya, Ph.D.

Part I

Bereavement, Grief, and Prolonged Grief Disorder: Clinical Presentations and Basics of Clinical Management

Stephen J. Cozza, M.D.
Joscelyn E. Fisher, Ph.D.

Stephen J. Cozza, M.D.
Christin M. Ogle, Ph.D.

Alana Iglewicz, M.D.
Abigail Clark, M.D., Ph.D.
Sidney Zisook, M.D.

Part II
Diagnosis and Assessment of Prolonged Grief Disorder

Part III
Treatment of Prolonged Grief Disorder

Contributors

Meredith E. Charney, Ph.D.
Clinical Psychologist, MaineHealth; Outpatient Psychiatry, Maine Medical Center, Portland, Maine

Abigail Clark, M.D., Ph.D.
Staff Psychiatrist, VA San Diego Health Care System, San Diego, California

Stephen J. Cozza, M.D.
Professor of Psychiatry and Pediatrics, Center for the Study of Traumatic Stress, Department of Psychiatry, Uniformed Services University of the Health Sciences, Bethesda, Maryland

Joscelyn E. Fisher, Ph.D.
Research Associate Professor, Center for the Study of Traumatic Stress, Department of Psychiatry, Uniformed Services University of the Health Sciences; Research Psychologist, Henry M. Jackson Foundation for the Advancement of Military Medicine, Bethesda, Maryland

Alana Iglewicz, M.D.
Associate Clinical Professor, University of California San Diego; Geriatrician, VA San Diego Health Care System, San Diego, California

Paul K. Maciejewski, Ph.D.
Associate Professor of Biostatistics in Radiology and in Medicine, Department of Radiology, Department of Medicine, Weill Cornell Medicine, Co-Director, Cornell Center for Research on End-of-Life Care, New York, New York

Christin M. Ogle, Ph.D.
Research Assistant Professor, Center for the Study of Traumatic Stress, Department of Psychiatry, Uniformed Services University of the Health

Sciences, Henry M. Jackson Foundation for the Advancement of Military Medicine, Inc., Bethesda, Maryland

Holly G. Prigerson, Ph.D.
Irving Sherwood Wright Professor of Geriatrics, Professor of Sociology in Medicine, Department of Medicine, Weill Cornell Medicine, Co-Director, Cornell Center for Research on End-of-Life Care, New York, New York

Charles F. Reynolds, III, M.D.
Professor in Geriatric Psychiatry, University of Pittsburgh School of Medicine; Professor of Behavioral and Community Health Sciences, University of Pittsburgh Graduate School of Public Health, Pittsburgh, Pennsylvania

M. Katherine Shear, M.D.
Marion K. Kenworthy Professor of Psychiatry, Columbia School of Social Work, Columbia University Vagelos College of Physicians and Surgeons; Director, Center for Prolonged Grief, New York, New York

Naomi M. Simon, M.D., M.Sc.
Director, Anxiety, Stress, and Prolonged Grief Program, NYU Langone; Professor, Department of Psychiatry, NYU Grossman School of Medicine, New York, New York

Natalia A. Skritskaya, Ph.D.
Adjunct Associate Research Scientist, Columbia School of Social Work; Clinical Psychologist, New York, New York

Sidney Zisook, M.D.
Distinguished Professor, University of California San Diego, San Diego, California

Foreword

The recent publication of diagnostic criteria and clinical diagnostic guidelines for prolonged grief disorder (PGD) in DSM-5-TR (American Psychiatric Association 2022) could not be more timely or important.

We find ourselves living in a global pandemic that has occasioned immense dislocation and disconnection: social, economic, political, medical, psychological, and spiritual. Our world has been turned upside down, perhaps nowhere more so than in Black and brown communities and, to our chagrin and shame, the United States as a whole.

In its wake, COVID-19 has wrought another pandemic of suffering, with pleomorphic expression: bereavement, acute grief, prolonged grief, depression, PTSD, substance misuse, and suicide. In addition, the ongoing epidemic of gun-related violence, particularly against children and older adults, greatly magnifies the occasions for loss and prolonged grief.

It is in this context that the editors of this handbook seek to offer science-based guidance to both the medical community and nonprofessionals. Our first goal is to help clinicians navigate the vicissitudes of typical ("normal") grief—that is, the process of adaptation to and acceptance of the finality of death—in their patients, their families, their colleagues, or themselves. Our second goal is to teach how to recognize when that process has been derailed. Under the latter circumstance, grief becomes prolonged, with an intense preoccupation with the loss as if it had occurred just yesterday. Grief and longing remain, with no relief in sight; rather, the individual continues to yearn for the lost loved one, to the exclusion of healing and getting on with life's journey. In the absence of a focused intervention, this state may last for months, years, or even decades. The failure to envision and restore a life of meaning without the loved one, together with profound suffering and impairment in major role functioning, constitutes the essence of prolonged grief disorder, as defined by new diagnostic criteria in DSM-5-TR and also embodied in ICD-11 (World Health Organization 2022).

This distinction between the journey of typical grief, on the one hand, and PGD (also called *complicated grief* in recent literature; preliminarily termed *persistent complex bereavement disorder* in section III of DSM-5 [American Psychiatric Association 2013]), on the other, is fundamental to the organization of this handbook.

As is now recognized by both the American Psychiatric Association and the World Health Organization, PGD does not represent, in any way, the "medicalization" of a "normal reaction" to the loss of a loved one. On the contrary, PGD has been adjudicated by the DSM-5-TR Steering Committee and American Psychiatric Association leaders to fulfill DSM-5 criteria for a mental disorder. This deliberation followed decades of considered research that amassed a large body of evidence supporting the need to recognize this distinctive condition. It can be diagnosed reliably and distinguished clearly from typical grief and co-occurring or preexisting disorders (such as major depression or PTSD). Most important of all, it can be successfully treated, not with the interventions for major depression or PTSD, but rather with a relatively brief but specific psychotherapy (PGD therapy, or PGDT). PGDT is theoretically grounded in models of attachment and contemporary understanding of emotional dysregulation; in addition, it addresses avoidant coping and counterfactual thinking.

Restating both the scientific and the ethical premise of this diagnosis and this handbook: The failure to recognize PGD puts the bereaved at risk, not so much for stigma (as "medicalization" critics contend), but rather for protracted suffering, poor physical health, social isolation, loneliness, shortened life expectancy, and suicide. Clinicians are now better able to accurately assess those living with prolonged grief, perform a differential diagnosis, and advise specific treatment that has established efficacy and safety. These tools are particularly important amid the COVID-19 pandemic and the epidemic of assault-weapon violence.

Within this framework, the editors have chosen to focus primarily on manifestations of grief, both typical and prolonged. To be sure, this handbook covers a lot of territory, including epidemiology, bereavement, theories of grief, circumstances of loss, life cycle considerations, and cultural issues. That being said, the central focus of the handbook is to present evidence-based approaches to assess typical and prolonged grief, together with strategies for the clinical management of typical grief (should that be necessary), data on specific treatment for PGD, and tips on when to refer for specialist care.

We acknowledge that, because the goals of a handbook are distinct from those of a textbook, our narrative is scientifically based and clinically relevant, but not encyclopedic. We are not offering a systematic review or a meta-analysis, although we have drawn on such literature. We offer citations to guide the interested reader to primary source material in such domains as epidemiology, neurobiology, nosology, clinical assessment, prevention, and treatment. We have sought to enrich the narrative through the use of illustrations, tables, and case examples (while protecting privileged health information). We conclude the handbook with a consideration of how to fortify oneself for the journey of grief and a brief heuristic analysis of needed research. Although there is much still to be done, we already know enough to be of real service to all those acutely grieving, those suffering with PGD, and the clinicians who care for them.

We hope that readers of this volume will share our enthusiasm that grief research has matured to the point where the bridging of science and service is possible. We thank our colleagues at American Psychiatric Association Publishing for their editorial guidance in preparing this handbook. Above all, we thank the subjects and participants in decades of National Institute of Mental Health–sponsored grief research, our partners in research and practice, to whom this volume is dedicated. Our hope is that this handbook will serve as a tool toward better self-care, care for colleagues and patients, and finally, diagnosis, treatment, and prevention of prolonged grief disorder.

Charles F. Reynolds, III, M.D.
Stephen J. Cozza, M.D.
Paul K. Maciejewski, Ph.D.
Holly G. Prigerson, Ph.D.
M. Katherine Shear, M.D.
Naomi M. Simon, M.D.
Sidney Zisook, M.D.
Natalia A. Skritskaya, Ph.D.
July 2022

References

American Psychiatric Association: Diagnostic and Statistical Manual of Mental Disorders, 5th Edition. Arlington, VA, American Psychiatric Association, 2013

American Psychiatric Association: Diagnostic and Statistical Manual of Mental Disorders, 5th Edition, Text Revision. Washington, DC, American Psychiatric Association, 2022

World Health Organization: International Statistical Classification of Diseases and Related Health Problems, 11th Revision. Geneva, World Health Organization, 2022

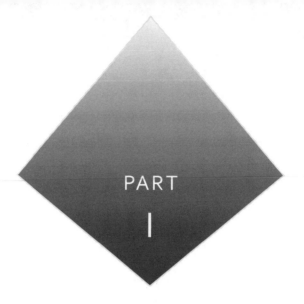

PART

I

Bereavement, Grief, and Prolonged Grief Disorder: Clinical Presentations and Basics of Clinical Management

Bereavement

Stephen J. Cozza, M.D.
Joscelyn E. Fisher, Ph.D.

Bereavement is a major life event, experienced by almost everyone throughout life. The word *bereavement* refers to "the objective situation of having lost someone significant through death" (Stroebe et al. 2008, p. 4). Bereavement typically leads to emotional suffering, particularly when it involves the death of a close loved one. The suffering, or what is referred to as *grief*, primarily involves emotional, but also physical, reactions to death (Stroebe et al. 2008). Although most who are bereaved adapt to the loss by incorporating it into their changed lives without the deceased, a minority experience long-term difficulties surrounding the loss that affect their mental and physical health. The goal of this chapter is to outline what is known about the epidemiology of bereavement and describe the experience of bereavement across the lifetime. This chapter also examines the effects of bereavement on mental and physical health outcomes and reviews the ways in which one may cope with the challenges associated with losing a loved one.

Case Example: Glenn

Glenn was 45 years old when he was diagnosed with pancreatic cancer. He was a well-liked and well-respected businessman who worked in a medium-sized company in Akron, Ohio, and served as an elder in his local church, where he sang in the choir. During his illness and his prolonged treatment that required trips to Cleveland for surgery and chemotherapy, he lived with Judy, his wife of 6 years, and their 5-year-old twin sons. Glenn also shared custody of his two teenage daughters with his first wife. Glenn was a member of a large extended family that was concentrated around Erie, Pennsyl-

3

vania. His 75-year-old mother was a cancer survivor herself and a widow who had lost her husband 2 years before Glenn was diagnosed. At Glenn's funeral were gathered 250 of his close friends and family members. His obituary stated that he was survived by his mother, his current wife and children, his two teenage daughters, three brothers, two sisters, multiple nieces and nephews, and countless cousins. His business partner, who was one of his closest friends, gave the eulogy, and the church choir sang at the funeral service. Afterward, Glenn's church installed a small fountain to memorialize him and the contributions he had made to their community.

Epidemiology of Bereavement

As illustrated in the above case example, a single death can impact many family members and friends. Nevertheless, the epidemiology of bereavement is difficult to comprehend, because most data collected within the United States and around the world are related to numbers of deaths, rather than the numbers bereaved by those deaths.

The top three causes of death across all ages in the United States are heart disease, cancer, and accidents (Heron 2021). In 2019, ischemic heart disease, stroke, and chronic obstructive pulmonary disease were the leading causes of death globally, accounting for 16%, 11%, and 6% of deaths, respectively (World Health Organization 2020). However, the leading causes of death shifted with the COVID-19 pandemic. Preliminary reports from the CDC (Ahmad et al. 2021) indicated that COVID-19 became the third leading cause of death in the United States in 2020, after heart disease and cancer, and it has been reported as the fourth leading cause of death worldwide (Troeger 2021).

Rates of death vary by sex. For example, data from the CDC National Center for Health Statistics show that age-adjusted rates of death in the United States were higher for males (846.7 per 100,000) than for females (715.2 per 100,000) in 2019 (Kaiser Family Foundation 2021a, 2021b; Population Reference Bureau 2002). Rates of death also vary by age. For example, all-cause infant mortality and early childhood illnesses account for elevated death rates during the first 4 years of life, but rates then decrease substantially until age 15, when they start to increase steadily with age (Kochanek et al. 2020). Causes of death also vary significantly depending on age. For example, deaths of younger people are more likely to be sudden and violent, whether unintentional or accidental deaths (the most common cause of death for all individuals younger than 45 years), suicide (the second leading cause of death for ages 10–34), or homicide (the third leading cause of death for ages 15–34) (National Vital Statistics System 2018).

National Center for Health Statistics data also show that age-adjusted rates of death vary by race and ethnicity. In 2019, age-adjusted death rates were highest in Black (870.7 per 100,000) and American Indian/Alaska Native (767.3 per 100,000) racial groups, followed by white (736.8 per 100,000), Hispanic (523.8 per 100,000), and Asian/Pacific Islander (384.9 per 100,000) groups (Kaiser Family Foundation 2021b). Some of the measured differences accorded to race and ethnicity in the United States have been attributed to inequities in access to health care and insurance, different rates of comorbid medical conditions, and varying exposure to traumatic events (e.g., violence, homicides, substance abuse) (Egede et al. 2012; Jackson et al. 2011; Schoenfeld et al. 2013). In addition, social factors such as low education, racial segregation, inadequate social support, individual- and area-level poverty, and income inequality have all been associated with elevated rates of death. The estimated number of deaths attributable to such social factors in 1980–2007 was comparable to the number of deaths resulting from illnesses and behaviors that create health risks (e.g., poor diet, physical inactivity) during that same time frame (Galea et al. 2011). During the COVID-19 pandemic, inequities were observed in cities such as New York, Philadelphia, and Chicago. Those communities with higher social vulnerability (or negative effects in the event of a disaster or disease outbreak) had COVID testing rates that were lower and positivity rates, confirmed case rates, and mortality rates that were higher (Bilal et al. 2021).

The complex relationships between age, sex, race/ethnicity, and the other noted contributors to mortality risk (e.g., poverty, inequities in access to health care) make it challenging to accurately determine the numbers of bereaved people in the general population, although older studies have estimated 1-year incidence rates of bereavement of first-degree relatives to be 5%–9% (Frost and Clayton 1977; Imboden et al. 1963; Pearlin and Lieberman 1979). An estimate has often been quoted of six individuals bereaved by each suicide; however, Cerel et al. (2014, 2019) questioned the evidence for such an estimate. In response to the lack of empirical information, they conceptualized a model that defined a range of proximity to a suicide event, including those *exposed* (who knew or identified with the deceased), *affected* (a subgroup of exposed who experienced significant psychological distress), and *bereaved* (who were most closely affected by the loss), whether short-term or long-term (Cerel et al. 2014). In a follow-up study using the framework, Cerel et al. (2019) concluded that a single suicide results in 135 exposed individuals; those affected or bereaved were estimated to be lower in number (not reported). Thus the authors concluded that suicide results in a greater number of bereaved individuals than previously proposed, many of whom may require supportive services and resources.

Similar calculations have been conducted to determine the numbers of bereaved individuals resulting from the recent COVID-19 pandemic. Using simulated kinship networks within race groups for different ages, Verdery et al. (2020) created an indicator of bereavement exposure—the COVID-19 bereavement multiplier—that estimated approximately nine close relatives (i.e., grandparent, parent, sibling, spouse, or child) bereaved by each COVID-19 death in the United States. These estimates varied slightly by race (i.e., white Americans, 8.86; Black Americans, 9.18) and by kinship to the deceased, with more individuals bereaved by the death of a grandparent, followed by death of a parent or sibling, and then death of a spouse or child. In addition, a bimodal distribution for ages of the bereaved was observed, with greater numbers of bereaved at ages 10–29 and 60–69 years (Verdery et al. 2020). Notably, using this bereavement multiplier of 9, and with current COVID deaths >1 million in the United States (as of March 2023), the number of COVID-bereaved Americans is estimated to be >9 million.

When estimating bereavement exposure more broadly, it is important to consider global differences in death rates and life expectancy (Mathers et al. 2017). For instance, data from 2019 indicate that in low-income countries, deaths by communicable diseases are more prevalent than elsewhere: the top causes of death were neonatal conditions, lower respiratory infections, and diarrheal diseases. Deaths from diarrheal diseases are also a concern in lower-middle-income countries, along with ischemic heart disease. Stroke and ischemic heart disease are the leading causes in upper-middle-income countries, where lung cancer and stomach cancer also account for a large number of deaths. In high-income countries, deaths from ischemic heart disease, stroke, and dementias such as Alzheimer's disease are the leading causes of death (World Health Organization 2020). More recent data indicate that COVID-19 death rates also differ internationally. Factors such as population density and rates of obesity and hypertension were identified as most strongly associated with differences in death rates among 30 industrialized countries (Gardiner et al. 2021).

In addition, life expectancy varies by country: Japan has the highest expectancy, at 84.3 years, and Lesotho the lowest, at 50.8 years. Life expectancy in the United States is 78.5 years (World Health Organization 2021). National differences in illness exposure, health care availability, and cultural attitudes about seeking care can create further confusion for those who are bereaved of loved ones around the world, as depicted in the following case example.

Case Example: Jawad

Jawad immigrated to the United States from Angola with his immediate family when he was 15 years old. The rest of his family (aunts, uncles, and cousins) remained in Angola. Over the years, Jawad kept in regular contact with one cousin, Arlyss, who was his age. They had a lot in common, with similar interests; they frequently joked about their family's escapades. Both married and had children and shared stories about their young families and their busy lives, and the two young men were in comparable physical health. At age 35, Jawad realized that it had been a few months since he had heard from Arlyss. He found out that Arlyss had been ill with tuberculosis, and his condition was not improving. Although Arlyss had started treatment, he had been embarrassed about the stigma in Angola surrounding TB and had discontinued the treatment. When Jawad found out later that Arlyss had died, he was saddened and confused. From his perspective, which was influenced by living in the United States where TB is not a health risk, he could not understand how someone so young and otherwise healthy could die from a treatable disease. Jawad felt guilty for not being able to aid his cousin before his death, and also for living in a country that afforded so many relative advantages.

Along with natural causes (e.g., disease), large natural disasters, including hurricanes, earthquakes, cyclones, heat waves, and floods, add to the numbers of those bereaved internationally, particularly in areas of the world with poorer infrastructure. Political violence causes bereavement throughout the world: Krause (2016) reported that political violence results in >500,000 adult and child deaths annually. Wars have resulted in millions of deaths—deaths in World War II alone are estimated at 60 million, including military personnel and civilians. Armed conflicts have contributed to a threefold increase in worldwide deaths since 2008 (International Institute for Strategic Studies 2019).

Similarly, human-caused mass casualty events, such as mass shootings, result in large numbers of bereaved individuals. Terrorist attacks—bombings, sarin attacks—occur worldwide. Some terrorist attacks have resulted in thousands of deaths, including the attacks of September 11, 2001, in which 2,996 people died.

Bereavement Across One's Lifetime

Loss during any time of life results in fluctuations of emotions and cognitions that evolve, typically leading to the integration of grief over one's lifetime. These emotions and cognitions can be reactivated by life events and experiences. For instance, a wedding or birth can reactivate memories of the deceased, temporarily increase a sense of loss, and bring emotional pain, as well as opportunities for further integration of the loss. Similarly, making new friendships, moving households, changing employment, entering psychotherapy, furthering education, and other life experiences all affect the integration of grief and loss across one's lifetime (McCoyd and Walter 2015).

Untimely Deaths

We are bereaved at different times during our lives, and the timing and causes of death can significantly affect bereavement responses in family members and friends. *Untimely deaths* (also called *off-time losses*; McCoyd and Walter 2015) occur at an unexpected life stage and sometimes when the bereaved is at an immature or developmental stage. Untimely deaths are also challenging because fewer peers may be available to serve as role models for those who are bereaved, or peers may distance themselves through unfamiliarity and discomfort with the loss. In addition, formal support resources may not be adequate because of the premature or unexpected nature of the death (McCoyd and Walter 2015).

Although the death of a loved one is never easy, some losses feel more "unnatural" than others. In the extreme case, the death of one's child is universally perceived as unnatural, an inconceivable experience for parents, who never expect to outlive their children.

Bereavement During Childhood

In general, a child is likely to struggle more with any loss than an adult because of developmental limitations. The experience of untimely parental death is especially challenging, because younger children depend on a caregiver and are cognitively and emotionally less able to comprehend or process the death. Bereaved children rely on surviving caregivers and other adults to help them cope with the resulting emotional and behavioral challenges. (See Chapter 2 for more details related to childhood bereavement and grief.)

Bereavement During Adolescence and Young Adulthood

Loss of a parent during adolescence may result in challenges to autonomy, identity formation, and relation formation. It is not uncommon, moreover, for a violent death—such as accidental deaths (e.g., motor vehicle accidents, fires, or home/office accidents), homicides, suicides, and deaths due to disaster, terrorism, and war—to be the first experience of bereavement in teenagers and young adults. One study on the prevalence of exposure to sudden and violent deaths in a nationally representative sample of adolescents found that 30% of teens had experienced such a loss by age 18, and that it was associated with negative academic and social consequences (Oosterhoff et al. 2018).

Bereavement During Middle Age

Loss during middle age poses unique challenges. Although the effect of parental loss during middle age is less well studied than during childhood, results suggest that the death of a parent is associated in older adults with decrements in multiple domains of psychological well-being, including mood, self-esteem, and substance use, as well as physical health. Those effects may be magnified along gender lines (e.g., the loss of a mother more difficult for a daughter and the loss of a father more difficult for a son) and are associated with the quality of the pre-death relationship with the parent (Marks et al. 2007). Perhaps because loss of a parent in midlife is perceived as less surprising and therefore less disruptive, bereaved adult children may feel that their loss goes unrecognized by others (McCoyd and Walter 2015). After the death of one parent, adult children often need to take on additional caregiving for the remaining, grieving parent, which may add to their responsibilities and possibly change their living arrangements.

Bereavement During Older Age

Older age is associated with multiple losses, including the deaths of lifelong friends, older relatives, and life partners, all of which can challenge one's sense of ego integrity and potentially lead to despair (Erikson 1950). Perhaps because of the pervasiveness of loss, older bereaved individuals may be more likely to feel that their grief is unacknowledged, as it is not unexpected and therefore may not be as actively validated by others. Health challenges in older age—whether one's own pre-existing illness or end-of-life caregiving responsibilities—can also be a burden after the loss of a life partner. Indeed, losing a life partner in older age is considered one of the most profound and life-changing human experiences (Carr et al. 2001) and can result in a loss of self-identity, daily routine, and social connection, even if only temporarily. Spousal loss is typically associated with a pervasive sense of loneliness, increased health-related concerns, and disrupted activities, all of which require a reworking of identity and reestablishment of social connections (Naef et al. 2013). Despite the pain associated with the death of a spouse in later life, there are opportunities to develop a sense of meaning and purpose:

coping strategies that acknowledge the loss through active grieving while maintaining a continued connection with the deceased, and restorative activities, such as problem-solving and social connectedness (Naef et al. 2013).

Bereavement Health Outcomes and Associated Risk Factors

Physical Conditions Associated With Bereavement

Bereavement is associated with certain physical and physiological health outcomes (for a review, see Ennis and Majid 2021), including increased immune, inflammatory, and neuroendocrine dysregulation (Cohen et al. 2015; Gerra et al. 2003; Irwin et al. 1987; Schultze-Florey et al. 2012), risk of major cardiovascular events (Buckley et al. 2010; Carey et al. 2014), increases in nonspecific somatic symptoms (Kowalski and Bondmass 2008; Morina and Emmelkamp 2012; Fisher et al. 2022; Stroebe et al. 2007), and (variably) risk of cancer (Jones et al. 1984; Lu et al. 2016).

Physical outcomes may also be influenced by the cause of death. For instance, a systematic review of studies that compared physical health conditions of bereavement found that those bereaved by suicide were more likely to experience pain, physical illness, and poor general health (Spillane et al. 2017) than those bereaved by other causes of death. Bereavement is also associated with mortality (for a review, see Stroebe et al. 2007), which varies by cause of death. For instance, those bereaved by cancer were not at elevated risk of mortality (King et al. 2013), but those bereaved by suicide were (Agerbo 2005).

Psychological Responses and Mental Health Conditions

Most individuals who lose a close friend or family member are likely to initially experience acute grief in response to the death. The intensity of this response typically diminishes over time as the individual adapts to the loss (Shear 2015). Importantly, acute grief is an expected response to the death of a close loved one and is not considered a clinical condition. As a result, no treatment is indicated for those who experience these symptoms within a year of a significant loss. Although the most common outcome following the loss of a loved one is resilience rather than pathology (Bonanno 2004), a minority of individuals (2%–3% worldwide) experience a longer duration of intense grief that impairs their daily functioning (Shear 2015). This grief-specific clinical condition is primarily characterized by persistent longing, yearning, or preoccupation with the deceased and has been variably referred to as complicated grief (Shear 2015), prolonged grief disorder (Prigerson et al. 2009), and persistent complex bereavement disorder (American Psychiatric Association 2013). Most recently, *prolonged grief disorder* (PGD) has become the accepted nomenclature for this condition, which has been formally included in DSM-5-TR (American Psychiatric Association 2022) and ICD-11 (World Health Organization 2022). See Chapter 4 for additional information.

In addition to typical grief reactions, bereaved individuals often experience symptoms of depression, PTSD, and anxiety that may meet a diagnostic threshold (Stroebe et al. 2007). For example, military widows are at increased risk for depression, PTSD, and adjustment disorder in the 2 years following a death compared with other military wives (Cozza et al. 2020). Correspondingly, depression, PTSD, and anxiety disorders are common comorbidities in those diagnosed with PGD (Simon et al. 2007). For instance, in a sample of bereaved parents, about half (49.5%) had elevated symptoms consistent with a diagnosis of PGD, and 59.1% and 74.9% had symptoms consistent with major depression and PTSD, respectively (Baumann et al. 2022).

Bereavement also carries a risk for suicidal ideation (Stroebe et al. 2005b), attempted suicide (Guldin et al. 2015, 2017), and death by suicide (Guldin et al. 2015, 2017). Although suicidal ideation is associated with bereavement in general, those bereaved by suicide are at the highest risk (Molina et al. 2019). In addition, PGD can elevate the risk for suicidality (Latham and Prigerson 2004; Mitchell et al. 2005).

The following case example describes the complex association of physical and mental health symptoms that can lead to suicide in those who are bereaved.

Case Example: Susan

Susan, age 53, met her husband, Bill, when she was 21. They felt a strong bond between them as soon as they met, which grew stronger over the years. They did everything together and raised two children. Once their children were adults and had children of their own, Susan and Bill enjoyed their ability to focus on each other again. One day, Bill went out to the store but never returned. A car had run a red light, crashing into Bill's car and killing him instantly. After this unimaginable event, Susan could not function. She felt as though her entire life and her identity had disappeared. Her kids were adults and she felt they didn't need her anymore, while Bill, her "soulmate," was gone. She developed persistent gastrointestinal bloating, cramping, and pain, as well as unexplained joint pain for which she was prescribed narcotic pain medication. One night, 4 months after Bill's death, when she was feeling particularly hopeless, Susan intentionally overdosed on her prescription pain medication.

Risk Factors for Poor Bereavement Outcomes

Given that the severity of the initial bereavement response predicts later ones, one study sought to identify individuals within 6 months of bereavement who may be at risk for manifesting multiple conditions during bereavement (Boelen and Lenferink 2020). Consistent with previous research (Cozza et al. 2019; Lenferink et al. 2017), three groups were identified: a low symptom group, an elevated grief group, and a group with high PGD, depression, and PTSD symptom scores. Compared with the two other groups, participants in the high symptom group were more likely to be female, relatively young, recently bereaved, and a partner or parent of the deceased, and the loved one's death was more likely to be unnatural. Participants in the high symptom group also endorsed a sense that the loss was "unreal"; had more negative cognitions about themselves, life, and the future; and had more avoidance tendencies.

The frequency and severity of problematic bereavement outcomes can depend on the circumstances of the death. For instance, sudden and violent deaths are associated with higher distress and more functional impairment, PTSD, and depression symptoms than nonviolent deaths (Green et al. 2001; Kaltman and Bonanno 2003; Kristensen et al. 2012). In addition, mass casualty events (natural disasters, terrorism, mass shootings, pandemics, or war) are often associated with PGD (Dyregrov et al. 2015; Johannesson et al. 2009; Shear et al. 2011), posttraumatic stress reactions, distress, and impaired general health in survivors (Dyregrov et al. 2015; Johannesson et al. 2009; Lowe et al. 2014). These individual effects of bereavement may be compounded by material losses—such as loss of home, income, stability, and sense of safety—given that neighbors and the local community may likewise have been affected. In addition, the high visibility (including media coverage) of these types of events can be a secondary stressor for the bereaved and is associated with higher rates of PGD (Kristensen et al. 2016).

Social Context of Bereavement

The social context of bereavement is critical to health and well-being as one deals with the aftermath of a death. Bereavement can lead to isolation and loneliness. Connections and involvement with family members, friends, communities, traditions, and religious rites can bring comfort. The sustained availability and palpable support of a network is protective to one who has suffered a loss. Although social support does not affect the impact of the loss, it can improve emotional well-being and reduce symptoms of depression (Stroebe et al. 2005c). Conversely, the type, amount, or timing of support can itself cause distress. It is important to ensure that the type of social support fits the bereaved individual's needs (Aoun et al. 2019).

Some factors can complicate a bereaved person's situation. For instance, quarantine restrictions resulting from the COVID-19 pandemic made it difficult, if not impossible, to participate in traditions, rites, and rituals that used to be typical after a death. Funeral services, memorials, wakes, shivas, and other observances were canceled or postponed, leading many to feel isolated and disconnected in their grief (Diolaiuti et al. 2021; Mayland et al. 2020; Stroebe and Schut 2021). In part because of such social disconnections, bereavement during the pandemic has been associated with more severe outcomes (Kokou-Kpolou et al. 2020).

Circumstances of the death may make it difficult for family members, friends, or others in the community to engage with the deceased. The cause of death may carry a stigma, such as suicide, murder-suicide, HIV/AIDS, and drug overdose (Brosnan 2013; Campbell 1999; Feigelman et al. 2011; Green and Grant 2008; Guy 2004; Valentine et al. 2016; Yamanaka 2015). Under those circumstances, bereaved individuals may feel uncomfortable engaging with others who might typically provide support for them, and those others may feel similarly uncomfortable, leading to a sense of disconnection and loneliness (Attig 2004; Brosnan 2013; Campbell 1999; Doka 1989; Feigelman et al. 2011; Valentine et al. 2016). In recognition of such circumstances, Doka (1989, p. 4) coined the term *disenfranchised grief* to describe "the grief that persons experience when they incur a loss that is not or cannot be openly acknowledged, publicly mourned, or socially supported." Disenfranchised grief leads to failures of empathy from individuals and communities that would typically offer support (Attig 2004; Doka 1989). The following case example provides an example of a loss that may go unrecognized or underappreciated.

Case Example: Chloe

Chloe, age 38, had been wanting a baby for years, but was unable to conceive. She and her husband decided to try fertility treatments, and after one cycle, she was excited to discover that she was finally pregnant. After the first trimester had passed, she started getting even more excited and began buying baby items and furniture to prepare for her little one's arrival. At 22 weeks' gestation, something didn't feel right to her, but she told herself she was being paranoid and waited a few days until her next doctor appointment. At that appointment, she was told that the baby's heart had stopped beating. "I'm sorry, your baby has died," they told her. "We have to deliver her." Chloe was devastated. She had to endure the physical pain of labor and the emotional pain of losing her baby. She and her husband, Kyle, held their tiny daughter, Hope, and said their goodbyes. Although they held a small memorial service for Hope, they did not share the news with many of their friends or co-workers. Several close family members who were invited did not attend. Chloe's brother, who did attend, asked her "Why are you making such a big deal about this? You need to get over it." Chloe returned to work shortly after the delivery. In the evenings, she would often cry, telling Kyle "Nobody cares. They all go on like everything is normal ... but it's not!"

Coping Following Bereavement and Associated Outcomes

Strategies for coping with stressful or traumatic experiences have been defined and classified in various ways in various populations (Carver et al. 1989; Lazarus and Folkman 1984; Parker and Endler 1992). Although the measurement of specific coping strategies and the labels for these strategies differ between studies, three similar coping dimensions have been identified (Gutiérrez et al. 2007; Hasking and Oei 2002; Litman 2006; Lyne and Roger 2000; Schnider et al. 2007; Wang et al. 2018): *problem-focused coping* (active coping, planning, using instrumental support, and engaging religion), *active emotional coping* (venting, positive reframing, using humor, employing acceptance, and engaging emotional support), and *avoidant emotional coping* (self-distracting, using denial, behavioral disengaging, self-blaming, and misusing substances). These coping strategies have been associated with specific health outcomes in bereaved individuals (Anderson et al. 2005; Drapeau et al. 2019; Harper et al. 2014; 2015; McDevitt-Murphy et al. 2021; Murphy et al. 2002, 2003a, 2003b; Schnider et al. 2007). For instance, problem-focused coping (Drapeau et al. 2019) has been associated with post-traumatic growth, and active coping has been associated with lower PTSD symptom scores (Murphy et al. 2003b). Avoidant coping has been associated with increased severity of negative outcomes, such as grief (Harper et al. 2014, 2015; McDevitt-Murphy et al. 2021), PTSD (Murphy et al. 2003a), mental distress (Murphy et al. 2002), and depression (Harper et al. 2015). It has also been associated with lower grief severity (Anderson et al. 2005), suggesting that the relationship between avoidant coping and grief severity is complex and likely affected by additional factors.

One factor is variability across time. Many studies have investigated coping strategies as static or fixed choices, when in actuality, a variety of coping strategies can be used by one person at any point in time, and several may change over time. The ability to alternate between types of coping, given that some coping styles are more useful than others at a given point in the coping process, has been referred to as *coping flexibility* (Bonanno et al. 2004). A similar perspective was outlined in the *dual-process model* (DPM) of coping with bereavement (Stroebe and Schut 1999, 2001). DPM suggests that while coping with bereavement, one oscillates between focusing on loss-oriented stressors (related to the loss itself) and restoration-oriented stressors (consequences of bereavement, such as rethinking or replanning aspects of one's life). However, Shear (2010) proposed that these processes may be better conceptualized as overlapping and occurring in tandem, rather than separate oscillating processes.

In addition to confronting versus avoiding loss- and restoration-oriented stressors, one may take a time-out and not engage at all. This variability within the timeline of coping is to be expected. Indeed, recently bereaved spouses reported experiencing positive emotions, including laughter, humor, and happiness, more often than they expected. Reports of high levels of these emotions were associated with lower levels of grief and depression (Lund et al. 2008). When oscillation between loss-oriented and restoration-oriented processes is absent, and one focuses on either loss- or restoration-oriented stressors to an extreme degree, problematic outcomes are likely to result (Stroebe and Schut 2010).

Thus, which coping strategies are used, how often they are used, and the timing of their use can affect mental health outcomes. For instance, avoidant coping (or experiential avoidance) can be adaptive immediately after the loss and may be used as a time-out, as mentioned above, but it can be harmful when used for a long period of time (Shear 2010). In fact, avoidance has been identified as a central aspect of PGD, in which avoidance of reminders of the loss is associated with functional impairment (Shear et al. 2007).

Continuing Bonds

After a death, continuing bonds—planning memorials, engaging with memories and images, in general keeping the deceased a part of one's life—is often a way to cope. However, the effects vary, which has led to debate as to whether it is better to maintain these bonds or loosen them (Neimeyer et al. 2006; Stroebe et al. 2005a). Attachment style may contribute to the effectiveness of continuing bonds. It has been suggested that securely attached individuals will react emotionally to the loss but not feel overwhelmed by grief, whereas those who are insecurely attached (preoccupied, dismissive, or disorganized) are likely to have more difficulty coping (Stroebe et al. 2005a).

Another factor that influences the effect of continuing bonds is meaning-making. If the bereaved individual is unable to make sense of the loss, stronger continuing bonds have been associated with more separation distress (Neimeyer et al. 2006).

Conclusion

Estimating the number of bereaved can be challenging, given that no existing data systems enumerate the individuals bereaved by the many deaths that occur each year in the United States and globally. Although many factors can affect estimates of the number of bereaved, several sources indicate that approximately nine close friends and relatives are manifestly affected by each death. The effects of bereavement differ across one's life span depending on one's age, one's relationship with the deceased, and the circumstances of death. Most bereaved people experience acute grief that dissipates as they integrate a new reality without their loved one. In some cases, physical illnesses, depression, anxiety, and clinically significant grief, or PGD, can follow bereavement, especially after sudden and violent deaths, mass casualty events, or losses that are considered disenfranchised. Bereaved individuals use a variety of coping strategies (such as continuing bonds), which are most adaptive when flexibly implemented over time. Longtime reliance on one coping strategy, especially avoidance, has been associated with poor bereavement outcomes, including PGD.

References

Agerbo E: Midlife suicide risk, partner's psychiatric illness, spouse and child bereavement by suicide or other modes of death: a gender specific study. J Epidemiol Community Health 59(5):407–412, 2005 15831691

Ahmad FB, Cisewski JA, Miniño A, Anderson RN: Provisional mortality data—United States, 2020. MWR Morb Mortal Wkly Rep 70(14):519–522, 2021

American Psychiatric Association: Diagnostic and Statistical Manual of Mental Disorders, 5th Edition. Arlington, VA, American Psychiatric Association, 2013

American Psychiatric Association: Diagnostic and Statistical Manual of Mental Disorders, 5th Edition, Text Revision. Washington, DC, American Psychiatric Association, 2022

Anderson MJ, Marwit SJ, Vandenberg B, Chibnall JT: Psychological and religious coping strategies of mothers bereaved by the sudden death of a child. Death Stud 29(9):811–826, 2005

Aoun SM, Breen LJ, Rumbold B, et al: Matching response to need: what makes social networks fit for providing bereavement support? PLoS One 14(3):e0213367, 2019 30845193

Attig T: Disenfranchised grief revisited: discounting hope and love. Omega (Westport) 49(3):197–215, 2004

Baumann I, Künzel J, Goldbeck L, et al: Prolonged grief, posttraumatic stress, and depression among bereaved parents: prevalence and response to an intervention program. Omega (Westport) 84(3):837–855, 2022

Bilal U, Tabb LP, Barber S, Diez Roux AV: Spatial inequities in COVID-19 testing, positivity, confirmed cases, and mortality in 3 US cities: an ecological study. Ann Intern Med 174(7):936–944, 2021 33780289

Boelen PA, Lenferink LIM: Symptoms of prolonged grief, posttraumatic stress, and depression in recently bereaved people: symptom profiles, predictive value, and cognitive behavioural correlates. Soc Psychiatry Psychiatr Epidemiol 55(6):765–777, 2020 31535165

Bonanno GA: Loss, trauma, and human resilience: have we underestimated the human capacity to thrive after extremely aversive events? Am Psychol 59(1):20–28, 2004 14736317

Bonanno GA, Papa A, Lalande K, et al: The importance of being flexible: the ability to both enhance and suppress emotional expression predicts long-term adjustment. Psychol Sci 15(7):482–487, 2004

Brosnan A: Stigmatized loss and suicide. 2013. Clinical research paper, St. Catherine University, 2013. Available at: https://sophia.stkate.edu/msw_papers/158. Accessed February 2, 2022.

Buckley T, McKinley S, Tofler G, Bartrop R: Cardiovascular risk in early bereavement: a literature review and proposed mechanisms. Int J Nurs Stud 47(2):229–238, 2010 19665709

Campbell T: AIDS-related death: a review of how bereaved gay men are affected. Couns Psychol Q 12(3):245–252, 1999

Carey IM, Shah SM, DeWilde S, et al: Increased risk of acute cardiovascular events after partner bereavement: a matched cohort study. JAMA Intern Med 174(4):598–605, 2014 24566983

Carr D, House JS, Wortman C, et al: Psychological adjustment to sudden and anticipated spousal loss among older widowed persons. J Gerontol B Psychol Sci Soc Sci 56(4):S237–S248, 2001 11445616

Carver CS, Scheier MF, Weintraub JK: Assessing coping strategies: a theoretically based approach. J Pers Soc Psychol 56(2):267–283, 1989 2926629

Cerel J, McIntosh JL, Neimeyer RA, et al: The continuum of "survivorship": definitional issues in the aftermath of suicide. Suicide Life Threat Behav 44(6):591–600, 2014

Cerel J, Brown MM, Maple M, et al: How many people are exposed to suicide? Not six. Suicide Life Threat Behav 49(2):529–534, 2019 29512876

Cohen M, Granger S, Fuller-Thomson E: The association between bereavement and biomarkers of inflammation. Behav Med 41(2):49–59, 2015 24266503

Cozza SJ, Fisher JE, Fetchet MA, et al: Patterns of comorbidity among bereaved family members 14 years after the September 11th, 2001, terrorist attacks. J Trauma Stress 32(4):526–535, 2019 31206211

Cozza SJ, Hefner KR, Fisher JE, et al: Mental health conditions in bereaved military service widows: a prospective, case-controlled, and longitudinal study. Depress Anxiety 37(1):45–53, 2020 31765052

Diolaiuti F, Marazziti D, Beatino MF, et al: Impact and consequences of COVID-19 pandemic on complicated grief and persistent complex bereavement disorder. Psychiatry Res 300:113916, 2021 33836468

Doka KJ (ed): Disenfranchised Grief: Recognizing Hidden Sorrow. Lexington, MA, Lexington Books, 1989

Drapeau CW, Lockman JD, Moore MM, Cerel J: Predictors of posttraumatic growth in adults bereaved by suicide. Crisis 40(3):196–202, 2019

Dyregrov K, Dyregrov A, Kristensen P: Traumatic bereavement and terror: the psychosocial impact on parents and siblings 1.5 years after the July 2011 terror killings in Norway. J Loss Trauma 20(6):556–576, 2015 21852658

Egede LE, Dismuke C, Echols C: Racial/ethnic disparities in mortality risk among US veterans with traumatic brain injury. Am J Public Health 102(S2):S266–S271, 2012

Ennis J, Majid U: "Death from a broken heart": a systematic review of the relationship between spousal bereavement and physical and physiological health outcomes. Death Stud 45(7):538–551, 2021 31535594

Erikson EH (ed): Childhood and Society. New York, W.W. Norton and Co., 1950

Feigelman W, Jordan JR, Gorman BS: Parental grief after a child's drug death compared to other death causes: investigating a greatly neglected bereavement population. Omega (Westport) 63(4):291–316, 2011 22010370

Fisher W, Krantz DS, Ogle CM: PMental health, ill-defined conditions, and health care utilization following bereavement: a prospective case-control study. J Acad Consult Liaison Psychiatry 63(5):434–444, 2022 35257945

Frost NR, Clayton PJ: Bereavement and psychiatric hospitalization. Arch Gen Psychiatry 34(10):1172–1175, 1977 911217

Galea S, Tracy M, Hoggatt KJ, et al: Estimated deaths attributable to social factors in the United States. Am J Public Health 101(8):1456–1465, 2011 21680937

Gardiner J, Oben J, Sutcliffe A: Obesity as a driver of international differences in COVID-19 death rates. Diabetes Obes Metab 23(7):1436–1470, 2021 33620765

Gerra G, Monti D, Panerai AE, et al: Long-term immune-endocrine effects of bereavement: relationships with anxiety levels and mood. Psychiatry Res 121(2):145–158, 2003 14656449

Green BL, Krupnick JL, Stockton P, et al: Psychological outcomes associated with traumatic loss in a sample of young women. Am Behav Sci 44(5):817–837, 2001

Green L, Grant V: "Gagged grief and beleaguered bereavements?" An analysis of multidisciplinary theory and research relating to same sex partnership bereavement. Sexualities 11(3):275–300, 2008

Guldin M-B, Li J, Pedersen HS, et al: Incidence of suicide among persons who had a parent who died during their childhood: a population-based cohort study. JAMA Psychiatry 72(12):1227–1234, 2015 26558351

Guldin M-B, Kjaersgaard MIS, Fenger-Grøn M, et al: Risk of suicide, deliberate self-harm and psychiatric illness after the loss of a close relative: a nationwide cohort study. World Psychiatry 16(2):193–199, 2017 28498584

Gutiérrez F, Peri JM, Torres X, et al: Three dimensions of coping and a look at their evolutionary origin. J Res Pers 41(5):1032–1053, 2007

Guy P: Bereavement through drug use: messages from research. Practice (Birm) 16(1):43–54, 2004

Harper M, O'Connor RC, O'Carroll RE: Factors associated with grief and depression following the loss of a child: a multivariate analysis. Psychol Health Med 19(3):247–252, 2014 23802736

Harper M, O'Connor RC, O'Carroll RE: The relative importance of avoidance and restoration-oriented stressors for grief and depression in bereaved parents. Psychol Health Med 20(8):906–915, 2015 25495761

Hasking PA, Oei TPS: Confirmatory factor analysis of the COPE questionnaire on community drinkers and an alcohol-dependent sample. J Stud Alcohol 63(5):631–640, 2002 12380860

Heron M: Deaths: leading causes for 2019. Natl Vital Stat Rep 7(9):1–114, 2021 34520342

Imboden JB, Canter A, Cluff L: Separation experiences and health records in a group of normal adults. Psychosom Med 25:433–440, 1963 14050425

International Institute for Strategic Studies (ed): The IISS Armed Conflict Survey 2015: The Worldwide Review of Political, Military and Humanitarian Trends in Current Conflicts. London, Routledge, 2019

Irwin M, Daniels M, Weiner H: Immune and neuroendocrine changes during bereavement. Psychiatr Clin North Am 10(3):449–465, 1987 3317313

Jackson JS, Hudson D, Kershaw K, et al: Discrimination, chronic stress, and mortality among black Americans: A life course framework, in International Handbook of Adult Mortality (International Handbooks of Population, Vol 2). Edited by Rogers RG, Crimmins EM. Dordrecht, Germany, Springer, 2011, pp 311–328

Johannesson KB, Lundin T, Hultman CM, et al: The effect of traumatic bereavement on tsunami-exposed survivors. J Trauma Stress 22(6):497–504, 2009 19937645

Jones DR, Goldblatt PO, Leon DA: Bereavement and cancer: some data on deaths of spouses from the longitudinal study of Office of Population Censuses and Surveys. Br Med J (Clin Res Ed) 289(6443):461–464, 1984 6432143

Kaiser Family Foundation: Number of Deaths per 100,000 Population by Gender, in State Health Facts. San Francisco, CA, Kaiser Family Foundation, 2021a. Available at: https://www.kff.org/other/state-indicator/death-rate-by-gender. Accessed December 6, 2021.

Kaiser Family Foundation: Number of Deaths per 100,000 Population by Race/Ethnicity, in State Health Facts. San Francisco, CA, Kaiser Family Foundation, 2021b. Available at: https://www.kff.org/other/state-indicator/death-rate-by-raceethnicity. Accessed December 6, 2021.

Kaltman S, Bonanno GA: Trauma and bereavement: examining the impact of sudden and violent deaths. J Anxiety Disord 17(2):131–147, 2003

King M, Vasanthan M, Petersen I, et al: Mortality and medical care after bereavement: a general practice cohort study. PLoS One 8(1):e52561, 2013 23372651

Kochanek KD, Xu J, Arias E: Mortality in the United States, 2019. NCHS Data Brief no. 395. Hyattsville, Maryland, National Center for Health Statistics, 2020

Kokou-Kpolou CK, Fernández-Alcántara M, Cénat JM: Prolonged grief related to COVID-19 deaths: do we have to fear a steep rise in traumatic and disenfranchised griefs? Psychol Trauma 12(S1):S94–S95, 2020 32525367

Kowalski SD, Bondmass MD: Physiological and psychological symptoms of grief in widows. Res Nurs Health 31(1):23–30, 2008 18161825

Krause K: From armed conflict to political violence: mapping & explaining conflict trends. Daedalus 145(4):113–126, 2016

Kristensen P, Weisæth L, Heir T: Bereavement and mental health after sudden and violent losses: a review. Psychiatry 75(1):76–97, 2012 22397543

Kristensen P, Dyregrov K, Dyregrov A, Heir T: Media exposure and prolonged grief: a study of bereaved parents and siblings after the 2011 Utøya Island terror attack. Psychol Trauma 8(6):661–667, 2016 27018922

Latham AE, Prigerson HG: Suicidality and bereavement: complicated grief as psychiatric disorder presenting greatest risk for suicidality. Suicide Life Threat Behav 34(4):350–362, 2004 15585457

Lazarus RS, Folkman S (eds): Stress, Appraisal, and Coping. New York, Springer, 1984

Lenferink LIM, de Keijser J, Smid GE, et al: Prolonged grief, depression, and posttraumatic stress in disaster-bereaved individuals: latent class analysis. Eur J Psychotraumatol 8(1):1298311, 2017 28451067

Litman JA: The COPE inventory: dimensionality and relationships with approach- and avoidance-motives and positive and negative traits. Pers Individ Dif 41(2):273–284, 2006

Lowe SR, Willis M, Rhodes JE: Health problems among low-income parents in the aftermath of Hurricane Katrina. Health Psychol 33(8):774–782, 2014 24295026

Lu D, Sundström K, Sparén P, et al: Bereavement is associated with an increased risk of HPV infection and cervical cancer: an epidemiological study in Sweden. Cancer Res 76(3):643–651, 2016 26634926

Lund DA, Utz R, Caserta MS, De Vries B: Humor, laughter, & happiness in the daily lives of recently bereaved spouses. Omega (Westport) 58(2):87–105, 2008 19227000

Lyne K, Roger D: A psychometric re-assessment of the COPE questionnaire. Pers Individ Dif 29(2):321–335, 2000

Marks NF, Jun H, Song J: Death of parents and adult psychological and physical well-being: a prospective U.S. national study. J Fam Issues 28(12):1611–1638, 2007 19212446

Mathers C, Stevens G, Hogan D, et al: Global and regional causes of death: Patterns and trends, 2000–15, in Disease Control Priorities: Improving Health and Reducing Poverty, 3rd Edition. Edited by Jamison DT, Gelband H, Horton S, et al. Washington, DC, The World Bank, 2017, pp 69–104

Mayland CR, Harding AJE, Preston N, Payne S: Supporting adults bereaved through COVID-19: a rapid review of the impact of previous pandemics on grief and bereavement. J Pain Symptom Manage 60(2):e33–e39, 2020 32416233

McCoyd JLM, Walter CA: Developmental perspectives on death and dying, and maturational losses, in Death, Dying, and Bereavement: Contemporary Perspectives, Institutions, and Practices. Edited by Stillion JM, Attig T. New York, Springer, 2015, pp 121–133

McDevitt-Murphy ME, Zakarian RJ, Luciano MT, et al: Alcohol use and coping in a cross-sectional study of African American homicide survivors. J Ethn Subst Abuse 20(1):135–150, 2021 31044649

Mitchell AM, Kim Y, Prigerson HG, Mortimer MK: Complicated grief and suicidal ideation in adult survivors of suicide. Suicide Life Threat Behav 35(5):498–506, 2005 16268767

Molina N, Viola M, Rogers M, et al: Suicidal ideation in bereavement: a systematic review. Behav Sci (Basel) 9(5):53, 2019 31091772

Morina N, Emmelkamp PMG: Health care utilization, somatic and mental health distress, and well-being among widowed and non-widowed female survivors of war. BMC Psychiatry 12:39, 2012 22578096

Murphy SA, Chung I-J, Johnson LC: Patterns of mental distress following the violent death of a child and predictors of change over time. Res Nurs Health 25(6):425–437, 2002 12424780

Murphy SA, Johnson C, Lohan J: The effectiveness of coping resources and strategies used by bereaved parents 1 and 5 years after the violent deaths of their children. Omega (Westport) 47(1):25–44, 2003a

Murphy SA, Johnson LC, Chung I-J, Beaton RD: The prevalence of PTSD following the violent death of a child and predictors of change 5 years later. J Trauma Stress 16(1):17–25, 2003b 12602648

Naef R, Ward R, Mahrer-Imhof R, Grande G: Characteristics of the bereavement experience of older persons after spousal loss: an integrative review. Int J Nurs Stud 50(8):1108–1121, 2013 23273923

National Vital Statistics System: 10 leading causes of death by age group, United States—2018. National Center for Health Statistics, CDC. Available at: https://www.cdc.gov/injury/wisqars/pdf/leading_causes_of_death_by_age_group_2018-508.pdf. Accessed December 1, 2021.

Neimeyer RA, Baldwin SA, Gillies J: Continuing bonds and reconstructing meaning: mitigating complications in bereavement. Death Stud 30(8):715–738, 2006 16972369

Oosterhoff B, Kaplow JB, Layne CM: Links between bereavement due to sudden death and academic functioning: results from a nationally representative sample of adolescents. Sch Psychol Q 33(3):372–380, 2018

Parker JDA, Endler NS: Coping with coping assessment: a critical review. Eur J Pers 6(5):321–344, 1992

Population Reference Bureau: The gender gap in U.S. mortality. December 1, 2002. Available at: https://www.prb.org/resources/the-gender-gap-in-u-s-mortality/. Accessed December 6, 2021.

Pearlin LI, Lieberman M: Social sources of emotional distress. Res Community Ment Health 1:217–248, 1979

Prigerson HG, Horowitz MJ, Jacobs SC, et al: Prolonged grief disorder: psychometric validation of criteria proposed for DSM-V and ICD-11. PLoS Med 6(8):e1000121, 2009 19652695

Schnider KR, Elhai JD, Gray MJ: Coping style use predicts posttraumatic stress and complicated grief symptom severity among college students reporting a traumatic loss. J Couns Psychol 54(3):344–350, 2007

Schoenfeld AJ, Belmont PJ Jr., See AA, et al: Patient demographics, insurance status, race, and ethnicity as predictors of morbidity and mortality after spine trauma: a study using the National Trauma Data Bank. Spine J 13(12):1766–1773, 2013 23623634

Schultze-Florey CR, Martínez-Maza O, Magpantay L, et al: When grief makes you sick: bereavement induced systemic inflammation is a question of genotype. Brain Behav Immun 26(7):1066–1071, 2012 22735772

Shear K, Monk T, Houck P, et al: An attachment-based model of complicated grief including the role of avoidance. Eur Arch Psychiatry Clin Neurosci 257(8):453–461, 2007 17629727

Shear MK: Exploring the role of experiential avoidance from the perspective of attachment theory and the dual process model. Omega (Westport) 61(4):357–369, 2010 21058614

Shear MK: Clinical practice. Complicated grief. N Engl J Med 372(2):153–160, 2015 25564898

Shear MK, McLaughlin KA, Ghesquiere A, et al: Complicated grief associated with Hurricane Katrina. Depress Anxiety 28(8):648–657, 2011 21796740

Simon NM, Shear KM, Thompson EH, et al: The prevalence and correlates of psychiatric comorbidity in individuals with complicated grief. Compr Psychiatry 48(5):395–399, 2007 17707245

Spillane A, Larkin C, Corcoran P, et al: Physical and psychosomatic health outcomes in people bereaved by suicide compared to people bereaved by other modes of death: a systematic review. BMC Public Health 17:939, 2017

Stroebe M, Schut H: The dual process model of coping with bereavement: rationale and description. Death Stud 23(3):197–224, 1999 10848151

Stroebe MS, Schut H: Meaning making in the dual process model of coping with bereavement, in Meaning Reconstruction & the Experience of Loss. Edited by Neimeyer RA. Washington, DC, American Psychological Association, 2001, pp 55–73

Stroebe M, Schut H: The dual process model of coping with bereavement: a decade on. Omega (Westport) 61(4):273–289, 2010 21058610

Stroebe M, Schut H: Bereavement in times of COVID-19: a review and theoretical framework. Omega (Westport) 82(3):500–522, 2021 33086903

Stroebe M, Schut H, Stroebe W: Attachment in coping with bereavement: a theoretical integration. Rev Gen Psychol 9(1):48–66, 2005a

Stroebe M, Stroebe W, Abakoumkin G: The broken heart: suicidal ideation in bereavement. Am J Psychiatry 162(11):2178–2180, 2005b 16263862

Stroebe M, Schut H, Stroebe W: Health outcomes of bereavement. Lancet 370(9603):1960–1973, 2007 18068517

Stroebe MS, Hansson RO, Schut H, Stroebe W (eds): Handbook of Bereavement Research and Practice: Advances in Theory and Intervention. Washington, DC, American Psychological Association, 2008

Stroebe W, Zech E, Stroebe MS, Abakoumkin G: Does social support help in bereavement? J Soc Clin Psychol 24(7):1030–1050, 2005c

Troeger C: Just how do deaths due to COVID-19 stack up? Think Global Health, September 22, 2021. Available at: https://www.thinkglobalhealth.org/article/just-how-do-deaths-due-covid-19-stack. Accessed December 7, 2021.

Valentine C, Bauld L, Walter T: Bereavement following substance misuse: a disenfranchised grief. Omega (Westport) 72(4):283–301, 2016

Verdery AM, Smith-Greenaway E, Margolis R, Daw J: Tracking the reach of COVID-19 kin loss with a bereavement multiplier applied to the United States. Proc Natl Acad Sci USA 117(30):17695–17701, 2020 32651279

Wang AW-T, Cheng C-P, Chang C-S, et al: Does the factor structure of the Brief COPE fit different types of traumatic events? A test of measurement invariance. Eur J Psychol Assess 34(3):162–173, 2018

World Health Organization: The top 10 causes of death. December 9, 2020. Available at: https://www.who.int/news-room/fact-sheets/detail/the-top-10-causes-of-death. Accessed November 2, 2021.

World Health Organization: International Statistical Classification of Diseases and Related Health Problems, 11th Revision. Geneva, World Health Organization, 2022

World Health Organization: Life expectancy at birth (years). Available at: https://www.who.int/data/gho/data/indicators/indicator-details/GHO/life-expectancy-at-birth-(years). Accessed November 2, 2021.

Yamanaka A: Japanese undergraduates' attitudes toward students survivors of parental suicide: a comparison with other stigmatized deaths. Omega (Westport) 71(1):82–91, 2015 26152028

2

Bereavement, Grief, and Prolonged Grief Disorder in Children and Adolescents

Stephen J. Cozza, M.D.
Christin M. Ogle, Ph.D.

Case Example: Joanne

Joanne, a 35-year-old single mother, worked as a nursing assistant at a community hospital in the Boston suburbs while earning her degree as a registered nurse by attending evening classes at a local college. She lived with her 11-year-old daughter, Brittany, who was a high-achieving sixth grader at a nearby public school. One November evening, while driving home from school, Joanne was rear-ended by a drunk driver, causing her to lose control of her car and crash into the highway median. She was killed instantly. Brittany's biological father had given up custody at birth, and his whereabouts were unknown. As a result, she moved in with her only known relative, her maternal grandmother, who lived in a rural community on the outskirts of Boise, Idaho. Brittany rejoined sixth grade in January at a local public school. New to the school, she was noted to be sullen and distracted, and her grades were mediocre. Over the years, Brittany increasingly argued with her grandmother, who was being treated for depression, chronic pain, and alcoholism. After dropping out of school at 16, Brittany moved in with her boyfriend's family and became pregnant with a little girl, Joan.

Children of all ages lose important loved ones, including parents, grandparents, siblings, and other relatives, as well as friends, teachers, and others. Despite their limited ability to communicate the pain of loss, children experience the same emotional, social, and physical consequences of grief as adults, but without the cognitive capacity and with greater interpersonal reliance on caregivers and other adults in support positions to help cope with the loss.

The main goal of this chapter is to provide clinicians with an understanding of how children experience bereavement and grief. Although many clinicians reading this text do not interface with children in their practices, they do treat adults who themselves have children that share their losses. This chapter is not intended to be an exhaustive examination of bereavement and grief in children, but a reference for clinicians to recognize that, like adults, children are powerfully affected by the deaths of loved ones in their lives. To address this goal, we provide a developmental perspective on grief and the unique challenges that children and adolescents face when bereaved. The chapter reviews the epidemiology of childhood bereavement, discusses the normative developmental responses to childhood bereavement and the mechanisms to support children under such circumstances, describes the current understanding of childhood *prolonged grief disorder* (PGD), highlights the developing evidence base for treating PGD in children, and provides the reader with additional resources that can assist in clinical practice.

Epidemiology of Childhood Bereavement

We know very little about the prevalence of childhood bereavement in the United States or globally. Despite the certain impact of loss during childhood, few mechanisms exist to measure the prevalence of bereavement among children. Although the numbers of adult and child deaths can be counted, the exact numbers of children affected by those deaths are unclear. Estimates of parental deaths have been proposed, however. For example, the United Nations International Children's Emergency Fund (UNICEF) estimated that nearly 140 million children worldwide experienced the death of one or both parents in 2015 (Burns et al. 2020). According to the U.S. Census Bureau (2014), more than 3% of children younger than age 18 in U.S. households were reported to have lost a parent in 2014, with more than three times as many U.S. children bereaved of fathers (2.37%) as mothers (0.78%). This proportional difference is because males of parenting age (18–44 years) are more likely than parenting-age females to die from causes both intentional (e.g., suicide, homicide) and unintentional (e.g., motor vehicle or occupational accidents) (Centers for Disease Control and Prevention 2017). Despite these statistics, more research has examined the effects of mother loss than father loss in children.

Burns et al. (2020) noted that the absence of a national tracking system to monitor childhood bereavement in the United States has made it difficult to accurately assess adverse outcomes related to parental and sibling loss during childhood. They introduced the Childhood Bereavement Estimation Model (CBEM), a quantitative statistical tool to more accurately estimate the numbers of children affected by such loss. They estimated that one in 14 children in the United States will experience the loss of a sibling or parent by age 18, and that rate is doubled by the age of 25 (Burns et al. 2020). Notably, the CBEM model predicts geographical variation in the prevalence of bereavement of parents and siblings within the first 18 years of life, with a prevalence as low as 4.9% in the District of Columbia and as high as 11.9% in West Virginia (see Figure 2–1) (Burns et al. 2020).

In addition to estimates of prevalence of bereavement of parents and siblings, Oosterhoff et al. (2018) reported results of a study examining first experienced sudden loss among U.S. adolescents who participated in the National Comorbidity Survey—Adolescent Supplement ($n=10,148$), a nationally representative sample of adolescents in the United States. The study examined responses to the question "Did someone very close to you ever die unexpectedly, for example, they were killed in an accident, murdered, committed suicide, or had a fatal heart attack at a young age?" They found that 30% of adolescents reported at least one such sudden loss by the age of 18, with the highest likelihood occurring at ages 15 and 16 (see Figure 2–2) (Oosterhoff et al. 2018). The authors also found that sudden loss was associated with "lower academic achievement, lower ability to concentrate and learn, less enjoyment of school, lower school belongingness, and lower beliefs that teachers treat youth fairly," even after adjusting for the effects of demographics and other traumatic exposures (Oosterhoff et al. 2018, p. 1).

COVID-19 deaths have added to the burden of childhood bereavement in the United States, with more than 140,000 U.S. children reported to have been orphaned since the start of the pandemic in early 2020 (Hillis et al. 2021). Hillis et al. (2021) reported that ~1.1 million children in the world suffered the death of at least one parent or grandparent from March 1, 2020, to April 30, 2021, with paternal loss being two to five times more common than maternal loss. Children's experiences of loss are likely to be accentuated by the multiple stressors they have experienced during the COVID pan-

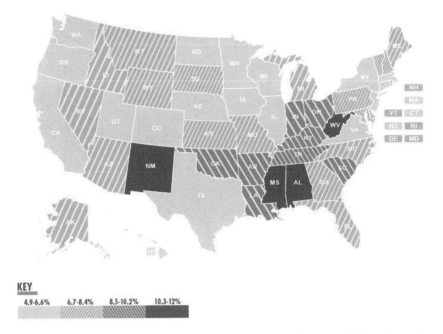

Figure 2–1.   Childhood Bereavement Estimation Model projected prevalance: variability by quartiles across the United States, percentage of children bereaved of a parent or sibling by age 18.

Data were extracted from the CDC Wide-Ranging ONline Data for Epidemiologic Research database for 2013–2017. Results reflect the average annual intercensal population estimates and the average annual death rates for that period.

Source.   From Burns M, Griese B, King S, Talmi A: "Childhood Bereavement: Understanding Prevalence and Related Adversity in the United States." *American Journal of Orthopsychiatry*, 90(4):391–405, 2020; used with permission of American Psychological Association – Journals, conveyed through Copyright Clearance Center, Inc.

demic, including the lack of connectivity with peers and other sources of support during required periods of quarantine and potential financial strain due to COVID-related job loss (Slomski 2021). Such experiences are exemplified in the following case example.

Case Example: Roberto

Roberto was a 17-year-old teenager who lived with his mother and grandmother in a suburb of Houston, Texas. He was a talented athlete who was a valued player on his high school baseball and football teams, and as a result, Roberto was connected to a broad group of friends with whom he enjoyed

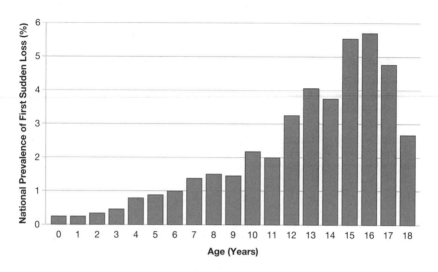

Figure 2–2. Prevalence of first sudden loss by age.

Estimates are weighted for ages 14–18 years to reflect the proportion of youth in the dataset at each age.

Source. From Oosterhoff B, Kaplow JB, Layne CM: Links between bereavement due to sudden death and academic functioning: results from a nationally representative sample of adolescents. *School Psychology Quarterly* 33(3):372–380, 2018; used with permission of American Psychological Association – Journals, conveyed through Copyright Clearance Center, Inc.

socializing. As a sophomore, his coaches were already talking about his potential to receive a scholarship for college athletics. Roberto was born in the United States, but his mother and grandmother were undocumented immigrants from Mexico. Given their concerns about increased surveillance by Immigration and Customs Enforcement, Roberto was encouraged to socialize outside his home, a modest two-bedroom apartment. After the start of the COVID-19 pandemic in 2020, Roberto's school quickly moved from in-person to virtual learning, and his connection with friends suffered. School athletic activities were canceled, and there were few opportunities for organized workouts with teammates. Roberto spent most days at home with his grandmother, as his mother was an employee at a local distribution warehouse where her job, the family's sole source of finances, required in-person work. His attention to schoolwork diminished, and his social interactions largely consisted of online gaming with friends that would often go into the early morning hours; as a result, his sleep schedule was unpredictable. In May 2020, Roberto's grandmother developed a cough that persisted for several days. Soon after, while Roberto's mother was at work, his grandmother developed a fever and she had difficulty breathing. Roberto reluctantly called 911, and his grandmother was quickly taken to a local hospital. He and his mother were unable to visit her. She died from COVID-19 after 2 days in the ICU. They never said goodbye. Although the extended family had met after other family deaths, no such opportunities were available during the quarantine. Roberto's mother encouraged him to stay connected to his grandmother, and to "talk" with her and with Jesus. However, he felt numb and disconnected. When he tried to imagine his grandmother, his memories of the sirens and EMTs entering their apartment on the night he called 911 were all he could recall. Sometimes he would have nightmares about EMTs coming back to the apartment to take his mother to the hospital. He felt utterly alone.

In addition to COVID, natural disasters, intentional acts of violence (e.g., school shootings, community violence), and acts of terrorism can result in child bereavement. For example, thousands of U.S. children lost parents and other family members in the September 11, 2001, terrorism attacks (Centers for Disease Control and Prevention 2002). During the 2011 earthquake and tsunami in Japan, an estimated 2,100 children lost one or both parents (Mie 2013). Political violence also significantly contributes to global childhood bereavement. The number of annual deaths due to armed conflicts has increased threefold since 2008 (International Institute for Strategic Studies 2019), and Krause (2016) reported an annual global death rate of more than 500,000 adults and children resulting from political violence. In addition, mothers and children make up the majority of victims who are displaced, traumatized, or killed in conflict areas (Save the Children 2014), underscoring the effects of traumatic loss on children around the world.

Mass shootings often occur in locations heavily frequented by children, such as schools, movie theaters, camps, and shopping malls, and as a result may be especially likely to result in bereaved children. For example, the 2011 mass shooting on Utoya Island in Norway took place at a youth summer camp. Of the nearly 70 people who died, the majority were children, who left behind bereaved siblings and classmates (Dyregrov et al. 2015; Strøm et al. 2016). Mass shooting incidents in educational settings accounted for nearly a quarter of all mass shooting incidents in the United States between 2000 and 2013 (Blair and Schweit 2014). The numbers of multiple-victim homicide incidents affecting U.S. children have been rising since 2009 (Frederique 2020), increasing children's exposures to the traumatic loss of friends and classmates. The challenges associated with childhood exposure to traumatic bereavement have been highlighted in the literature (Brown and Goodman 2005; Cohen et al. 2002) and are illustrated in the following case example.

Case Example: Minnie

Sarah and Minnie were neighbors and lifelong friends in tenth grade at their local high school. One afternoon after they had shared lunch in the school cafeteria, planned for an after-school get-together with other friends, and headed to their separate classes, a former student entered the school with a backpack filled with firearms. Although the school was alerted and classrooms sheltered in place, it took the police several minutes to arrive and subdue the shooter. During that time, he entered several classrooms, randomly shooting children and teachers, resulting in multiple injuries as well as three deaths, including Sarah. During the shooting, Minnie was hiding in the supply closet in the art room. After the shooter was detained, Minnie was unable to leave the room on her own, but was escorted out by the teacher and learned of the death of her close friend.

Throughout the next several weeks, Minnie was overwhelmed by grief, struggled with nightmares, and had difficulty returning to school, which was being held in an alternate location. She was often distracted in class, was reactive to loud noises, and described feeling "numb" much of the time. Although she attended the memorial service the school arranged for those who were killed during the shooting, Minnie was resistant to talking about Sarah or her death with the grief counselor that her parents arranged for her to see. In addition, Minnie avoided walking past Sarah's house on her way to school, taking an alternate, longer route.

Responses to Bereavement During Childhood and Adolescence

Normative grief reactions are expressed differently by girls versus boys and by children of different ages and developmental stages. A few studies have described sex differences in children's grief reactions following parental death. For example, bereaved daughters tend to evince greater internalizing problems (e.g., anxiety, depression) than bereaved sons (Raveis et al. 1999; Stikkelbroek et al. 2012, 2016), whereas bereaved boys have higher externalizing problems (e.g., hyperactivity-impulsivity, behavioral problems) than bereaved girls (Dowdney 2003; Dowdney et al. 1999; Rotheram-Borus et al. 2001). More information exists regarding differences in grief responses based on developmental age. Behavioral expressions of grief are likely more prevalent in younger children because their cognitive capacity is limitedand they lack the language skills needed to identify and report emotions. Research on developmental differences in bereavement outcomes described years after parental death indicates that bereavement in early childhood is associated with greater negative mental health outcomes than bereavement during adolescence (Berg et al. 2016; Pham et al. 2018; Wilcox et al. 2010).

Similarly, bereaved adolescents exhibit more intense grief reactions than bereaved adults (Servaty-Seib and Hayslip 2003). Here we discuss bereavement responses in children in different developmental stages.

Infancy and Early Childhood

Infants' and toddlers' experiences of grief are difficult to assess given their nascent language abilities and immature cognitive capacities. Children less than 2 years old are unable to understand death, being unable to engage in the abstract thinking required to process separations and loss. For example, a sufficient understanding of the concept of time, including a sense of past and future, is needed to help young children understand separations. Language skills, including sufficient vocabulary for emotion words, are also needed to help young children process the complex emotions often evoked by loss.

Nevertheless, it is important for clinicians to acknowledge that infants and toddlers experience grief, especially when associated with the loss of a primary caregiver. Their expressions of grief are similar to separation anxiety. Bereaved children under age 3 often protest the absence of their deceased caregiver by exhibiting waves of intense distress, despair, and anger. Responses to loss during early childhood may also be manifested as physical symptoms, such as stomachaches and changes in appetite. Young bereaved children also exhibit temporary regressions in the milestones specific to their developmental stage. Consistent and responsive caregiving can buffer bereaved young children from the adverse effects of parental death (Wardecker et al. 2017). Therefore, supporting the surviving caregivers' ability to provide these children with emotionally attuned, sensitive, and consistent care may help to promote young children's adjustment to loss of a parent.

Middle Childhood

Developmental advances in language, emotion identification and regulation skills, and symbolic thought facilitate school-age children's ability to understand and process interpersonal loss compared with children at younger developmental stages. Elementary school–age children's expressions of grief often entail periods of intense sadness mixed with periods of play. With age, children's abilities to modulate their emotional experiences grow, and they may adopt a preference for expressing their grief privately. Developmental advances in memory and abstract thinking also enable elementary school–age children to remember past experiences with their deceased loved one as well as imagine future events that will occur without the deceased. In general, these cognitive advances support children's ability to maintain a bond with the deceased, which is thought to facilitate their ability to cope with the loss.

Normand et al. (1996) proposed that children's connections with deceased parents typically follow standard progressions that evolve from conceiving of the deceased parent as a visiting ghost, to reliving memories of the past relationship with the parent and preserving personal belongings of the deceased parent as a link to the past, to maintaining an interactive relationship with the deceased parent by evoking the presence of the deceased throughout their everyday lives, to becoming a living legacy of the deceased parent by internalizing their values, goals, and behaviors. The starting point of an individual child's developmental progression through these ways of connecting with their deceased loved one depends on the age and developmental stage of the child when the loss occurred.

Adolescence

The continued development during adolescence of the prefrontal cortex, the area of the brain associated with problem-solving and judgment, allows for greater impulse control, more sophisticated social cognition, and more rational decision-making compared with younger children. These developmental advances coupled with increases in cognitive capacity enable adolescents to understand death and loss at a near-adult-like level. However, adolescents' emotional responses to death tend to involve cycling in and out of periods of intense sadness, similar to younger children. Over time, adolescents' expressions of grief become more similar to those of adults, which are characterized by preoccupation with the deceased, as well as periods of sadness and anhedonia.

Although adolescents have greater impulse control than younger children, their capacity to consider long-term consequences of their actions and fully control impulsive behavior is still immature relative to adults, which may lead to risk-taking behaviors. In addition, during adolescence, the asynchronous development of the amygdala and the prefrontal cortex, with the former developing earlier than the latter, promotes risk-taking behavior. Increased risk-taking behavior in this age group likely contributes to the high rates of death due to unintentional injury among adolescents and young adults. According to the CDC, unintentional injury and suicide were the first and second most common causes of death among 10- to 21-year-olds in the United States from 1999 to 2018 (Centers for Disease Control and Prevention 2019). The relatively high prevalence of death due to unintentional injury and suicide during adolescence renders this age group more likely to be bereaved by the death of peers and siblings compared with younger children.

After the death of a parent, adolescents are also more likely to inhibit their grief reactions to avoid burdening others, which often leads the surviving parent and other caring adults (e.g., teachers) to assume the child does not need support. In addition to intense feelings of sadness as exhibited by younger bereaved children, bereaved adolescents are more likely to experience fear and anxiety as they question the ability of the surviving members of the family to function without the deceased. In the context of this anxiety, parentally bereaved adolescents typically take on caregiving roles within the family (Cait 2005). If the surviving parent relies on the bereaved adolescent to provide care for younger siblings, the parentification of the bereaved adolescent may further interfere with the grieving process, as illustrated in the following case example.

Case Example: Jason

Jason was 16 years old and the eldest of three brothers living in the suburbs of Chicago when his 45-year-old father, Ken, died from colorectal cancer after a long and arduous treatment that included surgery, chemotherapy, and radiation. Although the family was prepared for Ken's death, the 4-year treatment had been especially fatiguing to Jason's mother, Barbara, who had accompanied Ken to most treatments and served as his main caregiver until his death. At the funeral, Jason's uncles reminded him that he was now the "man of the family" and needed to provide support to his mother and his brothers. During the months after the death, Barbara isolated herself in her bedroom and was unable to work or care for the boys. As a result, Jason took responsibility for many of the day-to-day chores in the house and for supervising his younger brothers. Although he maintained his grades, he spent less time with his friends, began to experiment with marijuana, and decided to skip tryouts for the school basketball team. Barbara contacted the school counselor to talk with Jason about his father's death; however, Jason refused to go, stating that he had too many other things to take care of rather than talking about his grief—"don't worry about me, I'll be fine."

The loss of a parent during adolescence, a period during which young people are typically striving to establish independence from the family, may result in disruptions in identity formation and the ability to establish strong peer relationships, including those with romantic partners. Parental bereavement during adolescence can also reduce adolescents' sense of belonging within their peer group (Hill et al. 2019). Compared with earlier phases of life, the death of a parent during adolescence is also more likely to impact youths' sense of economic security, career planning, and future academic goals, which can compound their vulnerability to long-term adverse psychosocial outcomes.

Clinicians need to recognize that the experience of bereavement in children and adolescents varies across developmental stages and often presents differently than in adults. An additional distinction between bereavement in children versus adults is that the former rely more on caring adults in their lives, whether they be parents, additional caregivers, or other trusted adults (e.g., teachers, coaches, or spiritual leaders), to help them regulate their emotions after a loss and orient to the new life created in the absence of the deceased. Although bereavement can lead to grief-related clinical outcomes, grief itself is neither pathological nor a disorder. As a result, when we consider interventions for bereaved children, we should emphasize supportive interactions that may benefit all of them. Kentor and Kaplow (2020, p. 889) summarized the evidence-based core components of grief-related interventions, which include "grief psychoeducation, building emotion identification and regulation skills, cognitive coping and restructuring, grief and trauma processing, memorializing and continuing bonds, meaning making, involvement of caregivers in grief treatment, and future planning." Although these components are important elements of treatments for grief-related disorders as described next, they also inform supportive interventions for any bereaved youth. Table 2–1 summarizes examples of typical expressions of grief during infancy, early childhood, middle childhood, and adolescence and provides examples of supportive actions that are helpful to children at different developmental ages.

When Clinical Assessment of Bereaved Youth Is Indicated

Clinicians must determine when children's grief responses are of a level that requires further assessment and potential clinical intervention. In addition to clinically relevant symptoms of depression, PTSD, anxiety disorder, or PGD, children's grief responses may include symptoms and circumstances that suggest the need for clinical assessment: suicidal ideation, physical symptoms with probable underlying psychological causes (e.g., headaches, stomachaches), academic problems, sleep problems or nightmares, changes in eating patterns, or loss of previously attained developmental skills (e.g., loss of bladder or bowel control). Children and adolescents that face unique circumstances may benefit from professional assistance after the loss of a loved one—for example, those who are traumatically bereaved (e.g., after suicide); those who are suffering from a serious, life-threatening, or termi-

Table 2–1.   Developmental expressions of grief and corresponding supportive actions

Group	Typical expressions of grief	Supportive actions
Infants and toddlers	Temporary developmental regressions (e.g., tantrums, dysregulation, clinginess, disruptions in sleep) Waves of intense distress, despair, and anger Physical symptoms (e.g., stomach aches, changes in appetite)	Maintain consistent routines Provide consistent, responsive caregiving Respond with empathy to children's distress (e.g., increased physical comforting, tolerance of and patience with regressive behaviors)
Preschool children	Temporary regressions in developmental milestones (e.g., bedwetting) Protests of the deceased's absence Fantasies about the deceased returning Nightmares Clinginess Symbolic play related to the death	Provide direct answers to questions about the death Clarify misunderstandings about causes of death (e.g., "this is not your fault," "you are not to blame") Clarify the permanence of death while focusing on ways to stay connected to the deceased (e.g., memories, photos, important possessions) Provide emotional support and model healthy grieving (e.g., acknowledge that loss makes us sad) Memorialize the deceased (e.g., talk about the deceased, draw pictures) Offer reassurance about the safety of the child and other loved ones
School-age children	Periods of intense sadness mixed with periods of play Preference for private expressions of grief Changes in eating and sleeping patterns Physical complaints Changes in academic performance	Encourage expressions of emotions about the death Provide developmentally appropriate explanations of the death Address fears about safety, illness, and injury with compassion and reassurance Address misconceptions about the death (e.g., guilt)

Table 2–1. Developmental expressions of grief and corresponding supportive actions *(continued)*

Group	Typical expressions of grief	Supportive actions
School-age children *(continued)*		Encourage opportunities to feel connected with the deceased (e.g., talk about the deceased, tell stories, memorialize) Encourage continuing healthy age-appropriate activities (e.g., school, involvement with friends, activities, sports)
Adolescents	Cycles of intense sadness, denial, and anger Social withdrawal Suicidal thoughts and thoughts of death Challenges connecting with others Inhibited expressions of emotion Difficulty concentrating Insomnia Risk-taking behavior	Emphasize the acceptability of differences in grief reactions Encourage opportunities to feel connected with the deceased (e.g., talk about the deceased, tell stories, memorialize) Address concerns about burdening others with their grief Address fears and anxiety about the ability of surviving family members to function without the deceased Encourage continuing healthy age-appropriate activities (e.g., school, involvement with friends, activities, sports)

nal illness; those with a prior history of emotional problems; and those with developmental disabilities. In such circumstances, children and adolescents should be referred to clinicians who are skilled in the assessment and treatment of pediatric bereavement (see Webb 2010).

Clinical Outcomes in Bereaved Children and Adolescents

The majority of research on grief in children has examined the effects of parent and sibling loss on children and adolescents, as well as peer loss during adolescence. Collectively, this work provides the foundation for our current understanding of clinical outcomes associated with childhood bereavement and grief. In addition to identifying resilience in bereaved children, this body of work also indicates that childhood bereavement can be associated with risk for a range of mental disorders, including anxiety, depression, PTSD, and substance abuse (Brent et al. 2009; Dowdney et al. 1999; Hamdan et al. 2013; Kaplow et al. 2010; McKay et al. 2021; Melhem et al. 2007, 2011). Bereaved youth have also been found to have higher risk of self-injury (Grenklo et al. 2013), suicide attempts (Feigelman et al. 2017; Kuramoto et al. 2010), suicidal ideation (Hill et al. 2019), delinquency (Feigelman et al. 2017), and violence (Wilcox et al. 2010), suggesting that parental death contributes to impulsivity, conduct disturbance, and aggression. Childhood bereavement has also been shown to negatively impact various aspects of youth academic functioning (Oosterhoff et al. 2018) and social development, including peer relations, career planning, and educational aspirations (Brent et al. 2012).

Although research associates childhood bereavement with mental disorders, longitudinal research on bereaved youth indicates that grief symptoms abate over time for the majority of children, irrespective of the cause of death (Melhem et al. 2011). Prospective research on young people's pre- and postloss mental health also indicates that mental health symptoms return to preloss levels within a few years after parental death. In a study of adolescents bereaved by HIV-related parental death, bereaved youth evinced elevated depression symptoms and impaired coping abilities following the death, but depression symptoms and coping abilities returned to prebereavement levels by 1 year after the death (Rotheram-Borus et al. 2005). Notably, a history of psychiatric disorders in children or family members before parental death increases risk for clinical disorders among bereaved youth (Brent et al. 2009; Melhem et al. 2008), suggesting that bereaved youth may benefit from clinical care to address preloss mental health disorders or intense grief reactions exacerbated by preloss disorders.

Like adults, for a minority of children, the loss of a loved one can result in prolonged and more severe grief reactions, in which case the newly defined DSM-5-TR (American Psychiatric Association 2022) clinical condition, PGD, should be a diagnostic consideration. Information regarding PGD in the pediatric population is summarized next, as well as information about treatment of children and adolescents with PGD. Like the traumatically bereaved adults who are more likely to meet criteria for both PGD and PTSD, persistent and severe childhood traumatic grief reactions occur among children who experience sudden, unexpected death caused by homicide or suicide, mass shootings, disasters, accidents, or sudden medical conditions. For example, a study of adolescents exposed to the sudden, violent death of multiple peers during a bus accident showed that the majority reported symptoms above the clinical cutoff for probable PTSD 18 months after the accident, irrespective of physical proximity to the event or psychological proximity to the deceased (Giannopoulou et al. 2021). *Childhood traumatic grief* (CTG) has been proposed as a clinical condition to describe the intrusive and distressing traumatic thoughts and memories that complicate the child's normative capacity to grieve and integrate traumatic losses (Cohen et al. 2002, 2006). Although CTG has been described as a unique disorder, distinct from uncomplicated bereavement, PTSD, and PGD (Cohen et al. 2006), and for which a specific cognitive-behavioral therapy has been described (CBT-CTG; Cohen and Mannarino 2004), it is currently not a recognized disorder in DSM. As a result, both PGD and PTSD would be indicated DSM diagnoses for traumatically bereaved children who present with a constellation of grief and trauma symptoms.

Risk factors contributing to more problematic grief-related outcomes have also been examined in children and adolescents. For example, the risk of adverse outcomes is higher among younger bereaved children compared with adolescents (Berg et al. 2016; Pham et al. 2018; Wilcox et al. 2010) and among bereaved children in families of lower socioeconomic status (Cerel et al. 2006; Kalantari and Vostanis 2010). More severe childhood grief reactions to parental deaths have also been consistently associated with poorer well-being in the remaining caregiver (Cerel et al. 2006), which illustrates the interrelationship of child and parent grief responses. Studies examining grief reactions consistent with childhood PGD identify female sex, prior exposure to interpersonal conflict, a history of depression or anxiety disorder, and parental bereavement that results from a protracted condition, in addition to traumatic loss, as risk factors.

In contrast to the well-documented effects of childhood parental bereavement on psychiatric morbidity, relatively few studies have examined physical health outcomes associated with childhood bereavement. However, the documented increase in all-cause mortality among adults with histories of childhood parental (Li et al. 2014) and sibling (Yu et al. 2017) death indicates that childhood bereavement may have long-term effects on physical health beyond its more immediate impact on mental health and well-being. One mechanism proposed to link childhood bereavement to adverse physical health outcomes involves disruptions in biological stress response systems, which is supported by evidence of dysregulated hypothalamic-pituitary-adrenal (HPA) axis activity in individuals with histories of childhood parental bereavement compared with individuals not affected by parental bereavement (Nicolson 2004). Obesity is another potential mechanism linking childhood bereavement to heightened risk of adverse health outcomes. In a prospective examination of parentally bereaved and nonbereaved youth, bereaved youth were more likely to have a body mass index in the obese range 5 years after the death (Weinberg et al. 2013).

PGD in Children and Adolescents

Case Example: Allison

Allison was 12 years old when her mother, Teresa, died after a 7-year battle with metastatic breast cancer. Teresa had previously been an extremely active adult who enjoyed running, hiking, and gardening. In addition, she had been Allison's primary caregiver, as she had decided to take a hiatus from her job as an attorney and be home with her growing family. Although many photographs of Teresa showed her playing with Allison and her siblings and being involved in many activities and celebrations, a testament to her prior health, by the time of Teresa's death these photographs seemed to be of a different person. Teresa was often resting in bed due to fatigue from chemotherapy treatments and, as death approached, bone pain resulting from the cancer's spread. A month before Teresa's death, Allison was awakened in the middle of the night by her father's frantic cries. When she entered her parents' bedroom Allison witnessed her mother's generalized seizure that was followed quickly by the entry of a paramedic team that took Teresa to the hospital. In the stillness of the house after her mother's departure, Allison worried that she would never see her mother again. However, Teresa did return and received end-of-life home hospice care.

After Teresa's death, Allison grieved in ways that her family felt were typical for a girl who had lost her mother. However, when Allison continued to show signs of depression, tearfulness, and nightmares and voiced thoughts that she no longer wanted to live, her father consulted a mental health provider. In those sessions, Allison reported tremendous sadness about her mother's death, a longing to be with her, and a lack of purpose in life. The memories Allison could conjure of her mother were only when she was extremely ill and suffering. A sense of anger and horror occurred when such images intruded on images of her mother when she was healthy. "She always smelled sick. I remember when I tried to kiss her, her breath was so bad that I had to leave the room."

As this case example illustrates, children, like adults, can suffer from PGD, a clinical condition that occurs in a minority of bereaved individuals. PGD includes prolonged and intense grief, persistent longing for the deceased, preoccupation about the deceased and how they died, and difficulty accepting the death, as well as other associated symptoms such as anger and bitterness, avoidance of reminders of the deceased, and suicidal thoughts, all of which contribute to distress and functional impairment (Melhem et al.

2011). Although PGD is now a diagnosable condition in children and adolescents, the disorder in the pediatric population remains less well researched than in adults. The progression of terminology from *traumatic grief* to *complicated grief* to *persistent complex bereavement disorder* to PGD, along with iterations of recommended criteria to diagnose such a condition and the need to develop assessment instruments for use in the pediatric population, has slowed the advancement of knowledge in this area. In addition, developmental differences in how PGD symptoms are expressed among children of different ages add further complexity to how PGD should be defined, assessed, and potentially treated in children of different ages. Nevertheless, clinicians should be aware of the important work that has been done in examining PGD in children and adolescents, including what we know about its phenomenology, assessment, and treatment.

The first discussion of clinically impairing grief in children focused on traumatic grief in the 1990s (Nader 1997) and was further outlined after the events of September 11, 2001 (Brown and Goodman 2005; Cohen and Mannarino 2004). Although much clinical and research interest was initially focused on a childhood disorder involving traumatic exposure to death, other researchers incorporated knowledge from the adult literature on grief to describe what has come to be referred to as childhood PGD (Melhem et al. 2004). Melhem et al. (2004) described PGD in children as similar to that of adults and focused on a cluster of grief-specific symptoms, such as yearning for and preoccupation with the deceased, as well as symptoms of distress (e.g., crying). Although the researchers found that childhood PGD was often comorbid with depression and PTSD, grief-specific symptoms were distinctly associated with functional impairment, poor adjustment, and suicidal ideation (Melhem et al. 2004, 2008, 2011). This complex and comorbid relationship between PGD, depression, and PTSD in bereaved children and adolescents has been reported by other authors (Boelen et al. 2017; Claycomb et al. 2016), all of whom have similarly identified childhood PGD as a distinct clinical condition.

The results of the few studies that have informed our understanding of the prevalence of PGD in children should be considered preliminary given that samples were not representative of all bereaved children. For example, in a study in which trajectories of grief reactions were observed in children and adolescents bereaved by sudden parental death, Melhem et al. (2011) identified three trajectories of grief reactions, with more than half of participants reporting rapid resolution of grief symptoms, 31%, a more gradual reduction in grief, and 10% endorsing sustained and prolonged grief symptoms 3 years after the death. Boelen et al. (2019) estimated a similar prevalence of probable PGD, 3.4%–12.4%, in a sample of help-seeking 8- to 18-year-old bereaved children, depending on the diagnostic criteria used. Further studies are required of PGD prevalence in large groups of children of different ages and bereaved of different relations by varying causes.

The final approved DSM criteria for PGD require that children and adults meet similar requirements to be diagnosed with the disorder. Although DSM does not currently identify a developmental subtype of PGD, as it does for PTSD, there has been thoughtful attention to developmental considerations in applying PGD diagnostic criteria to children. For example, Kaplow et al. (2012, p. 250) suggested a reduction of the 12-month symptom requirement to 6 months for children. In addition, they suggested a modification to the then-proposed criteria, such that "[m]ourning shows substantial cultural *and developmental* variation; the bereavement reaction must be out of proportion or inconsistent with cultural, religious, *or age-appropriate* norms" [proposed additions set as italics in original]. They also proposed that symptom requirements in children "may be expressed in play and behavior," that difficulty accepting the death may depend upon a child's "capacity to understand the nature and permanence of death," and that avoidance of reminders of the loss include "avoidance of thoughts and feelings regarding the deceased" (Kaplow et al. 2012, p. 245). More recently, Kentor and Kaplow (2020) offered a more comprehensive description of what developmental issues clinicians should consider when applying DSM criteria for PGD in children. For example, children may demonstrate preoccupation with the person who died by "sleeping in the parent's bed, or wearing their clothing or jewelry" (p. 890). Clinicians should pay careful attention to how children express symptoms of grief differently than adults and incorporate that understanding into their diagnostic considerations.

A comprehensive clinical assessment using the newly defined DSM criteria that reflects developmental symptomatology in children is the most effective method to identify PGD in the pediatric population. Although assessment instruments can be helpful, most that assess PGD in children have been developed for research purposes, and only some have incorporated developmental principles. For example, Melhem et al. (2007, 2011) presented the psychometric properties of the Inventory of Complicated Grief—Revised for Children (ICG-R or ICG-RC), a modified version of the original ICG (Prigerson et al. 1995), which they found to be a reliable measure of PGD, possessing internal consistency and convergent and discriminant validity. The psychometric properties of the Inventory of Prolonged Grief for Children (IPG-C) and the Inventory of Prolonged Grief for Adolescents (IPG-A) were described by Spuij et al. (2012) to include their concurrent, convergent and divergent, and incremental validity. Kaplow et al. (2018) reported the convergent, discriminant, and discriminant-groups validity, as well as the developmental and clinical utility, of the Persistent Complex Bereavement Disorder (PCBD) Checklist, an instrument that was based on a former version of the DSM PGD criteria, and that was developmentally tailored. The use of these assessment instruments for assessing childhood PGD in the clinical setting may be helpful, but requires further guidance.

Evidence-Based Grief Treatments

When children and adolescents are bereaved of loved ones, one should anticipate a broad range of grief responses. Most will reflect a normative and developmentally varying capacity to manage the loss, but others will struggle with adaptation, and a smaller group will have grief severity and associated grief-related symptoms that require clinical attention. Most children will benefit from the kinds of support that are outlined in Table 2–1. However, clinicians must be able to distinguish the majority of children who benefit from supportive interventions from those who evidence pathological grief responses, such as PGD, and who require evidence-based treatment. Although multiple interventions for bereaved children have been described in the literature, they have varied in their focus on support versus treatment and in the scientific rigor with which they have been assessed. Here we briefly summarize the few that have relevance to the treatment of grief-related clinical disorders (i.e., PGD) and that have been assessed in at least one randomized controlled trial (RCT).

The *Family Bereavement Program* (FBP) is the most studied program for bereaved children and has shown long-term improvements in bereaved children's self-esteem, internalizing and externalizing problems (Sandler et al. 2010a), suicidal ideation and attempts (Sandler et al. 2016), and levels of problematic grief (Sandler et al. 2010b) in RCTs. FBP is a 12-session preventive intervention for parentally bereaved children and their adult caregivers designed to educate them about the grief process and allow them to acquire and practice skills that promote child- and family-related resilience and prevent grief-related mental health complications (Sandler et al. 2013). Although structured as a preventive intervention, FBP clearly has clinical implications; however, further study of its effects within clinical populations with diagnosed PGD is required. Thurman et al. (2017) reported the positive effects of *Abangane*, an eight-session, locally derived, and culturally attuned supportive intervention for parentally bereaved female adolescents in a waitlist-controlled RCT. Although intervention effects on problematic grief and depression were promising, further study within clinical populations with PGD in an active-control RCT is required.

Two additional RCTs examined treatment effects within bereaved child and adolescent populations with identified grief-related clinical disorders. Layne et al. (2008) reported the benefits of *Trauma and Grief Component Therapy* (TGCT), a classroom-based intervention and 17-session group therapy including four developmentally informed modules addressing trauma and grief. TGCT reduced maladaptive grief reactions in an RCT that included 127 war-exposed adolescents with clinically impairing conditions, including depression, PTSD, or maladaptive grief (Layne et al. 2008). Although the study was conducted before diagnostic criteria for PGD were included in DSM, study results indicate its likely benefit for those affected by this disorder. More recently, Boelen et al. (2021) reported the results of the only RCT to date of bereaved children and adolescents diagnosed using a reliable instrument measuring childhood PGD. *CBT Grief-Help*, a CBT specifically designed to treat PGD in children and adolescents, is a manualized treatment that includes nine sessions for bereaved children and five parent guidance sessions. The intervention targets insufficient integration of the loss, rigid negative thinking about oneself and the world, and anxious avoidance by using psychoeducation, skill-building, and imaginary and in vivo exposures. In comparison with a group who received supportive counseling alone, CBT Grief-Help participants were shown to have continued improvement 6 and 12 months after treatment in symptoms of PGD, depression, PTSD, and other internalizing problems (Boelen et al. 2021).

Clinicians should note that there are no established indications for the use of psychopharmacotherapy in the treatment of childhood grief-related clinical conditions. However, medication should be considered to treat comorbid anxiety and depression or to assist with sleep, when indicated.

Conclusion

This chapter describes the challenges that children and adolescents face when bereaved, as well as the normative developmental responses to childhood bereavement. Although bereaved youth may be limited in their cognitive capacity to understand the finality of death and to communicate the pain of loss, they often suffer the same emotional, social, and physical consequences of grief as adults, but with greater interpersonal reliance on caregivers and other supportive adults to help cope with the loss. Grief symptoms typically abate within a few years for the majority of children irrespective of the cause of death. However, factors that increase children's risk of clinical impairment should be considered, including a history of depression or anxiety disorder, parental bereavement that results from protracted medical conditions, and traumatic loss. In addition, some symptom presentations may require further clinical assessment, including suicidal ideation, physical symptoms with probable underlying psychological causes (e.g., headaches, stomachaches), and severe sleep problems.

Clinicians need to be aware that a minority of bereaved children can be afflicted with a newly defined DSM condition, PGD. Core symptoms associated with this disorder include prolonged and intense grief symptoms associated with longing for the deceased, preoccupation with the deceased and how they died, and additional grief-related symptoms that may manifest in various ways depending on children's developmental capacity. PGD in children is associated with heightened distress and functional impairment, is often comorbid with other mental disorders (e.g., depression, PTSD), and, as in adults, responds to grief-specific evidence-based treatments. Clinicians should be prepared to assess bereaved children for PGD and other grief-related conditions and, when appropriate, refer them to competent services that offer evidence-based treatments. The newly defined DSM diagnostic criteria for childhood PGD will facilitate future research regarding PGD within the pediatric population and will inform our understanding of its prevalence and developmental variance among bereaved children, as well as its response to proposed treatments.

Resources

American Academy of Child and Adolescent Psychiatry (AACAP) resources on grief in childhood: https://www.aacap.org/AACAP/Families_and_Youth/Facts_for_Families/FFF-Guide/Children-And-Grief-008.aspx

American Academy of Pediatrics (AAP) resources on childhood grief: https://www.healthychildren.org/English/healthy-living/emotional-wellness/Building-Resilience/Pages/Grieving-Whats-Normal-When-to-Worry.aspx

Children's Bereavement Center resources: https://childbereavement.org/resources/

Doug Center resources on child, teen, and family grief: https://www.dougy.org/

Lieberman AF, Compton NC, Van Horn P, Ippen CG: Losing a Parent to Death in the Early Years: Guidelines for the Treatment of Traumatic Bereavement in Infancy and Early Childhood. Washington, DC, ZERO TO THREE/National Center for Infants, Toddlers and Families, 2003

National Alliance for Children's Grief resources: https://childrengrieve.org/

National Child Traumatic Stress Network (NCTSN) resources on childhood traumatic grief: https://www.nctsn.org/what-is-child-trauma/trauma-types/traumatic-grief

National Child Traumatic Stress Network (NCTSN) resources on COVID-related
childhood grief: https://www.nctsn.org/sites/default/files/resources/fact-sheet/
helping_children_with_traumatic_separation_or_traumatic_grief_related_to_
covid19.pdf

Sesame Workshop resources on childhood grief:
https://sesamestreetincommunities.org/topics/grief/

Webb NB (ed): Helping Bereaved Children: A Handbook for Practitioners, 3rd Edition. New York, Guilford Press, 2010

References

American Psychiatric Association: Diagnostic and Statistical Manual of Mental Disorders, 5th Edition, Text Revision. Washington, DC, American Psychiatric Association, 2022

Berg L, Rostila M, Hjern A: Parental death during childhood and depression in young adults—a national cohort study. J Child Psychol Psychiatry 57(9):1092–1098, 2016 27058980

Blair JP, Schweit KW: A Study of Active Shooter Incidents, 2000–2013. Washington, DC, Texas State University and Federal Bureau of Investigation, U.S. Department of Justice, 2014

Boelen PA, Spuij M, Reijntjes AHA: Prolonged grief and posttraumatic stress in bereaved children: a latent class analysis. Psychiatry Res 258:518–524, 2017 28958457

Boelen PA, Spuij M, Lenferink LIM: Comparison of DSM-5 criteria for persistent complex bereavement disorder and ICD-11 criteria for prolonged grief disorder in help-seeking bereaved children. J Affect Disord 250:71–78, 2019 30836282

Boelen PA, Lenferink LIM, Spuij M: CBT for prolonged grief in children and adolescents: a randomized clinical trial. Am J Psychiatry 178(4):294–304, 2021 33472391

Brent D, Melhem N, Donohoe MB, Walker M: The incidence and course of depression in bereaved youth 21 months after the loss of a parent to suicide, accident, or sudden natural death. Am J Psychiatry 166(7):786–794, 2009 19411367

Brent DA, Melhem NM, Masten AS, et al: Longitudinal effects of parental bereavement on adolescent developmental competence. J Clin Child Adolesc Psychol 41(6):778–791, 2012 23009724

Brown EJ, Goodman, RF: Childhood traumatic grief: an exploration of the construct in children bereaved on September 11. J Clin Child Adolesc Psychol 34(2):248–259, 2005 15901225

Burns M, Griese B, King S, Talmi A: Childhood bereavement: understanding prevalence and related adversity in the United States. Am J Orthopsychiatry 90(4):391–405, 2020 31999137

Cait C-A: Parental death, shifting family dynamics, and female identity development. Omega (Westport) 51(2):87–105, 2005

Centers for Disease Control and Prevention: Injuries and illnesses among New York City Fire Department rescue workers after responding to the World Trade Center attacks. MMWR Morb Mortal Wkly Rep 51:1–5, 2002

Centers for Disease Control and Prevention: Underlying cause of death. Unpublished raw data, 2017. Available at: https://wonder.cdc.gov/. Accessed December 1, 2021

Centers for Disease Control and Prevention: WISQARS™ – Web-based Injury Statistics Query and Reporting System. Unpublished raw data, 2019. Available at: https://www.cdc.gov/injury/wisqars/index.html. Accessed December 1, 2021

Cerel J, Fristad MA, Verducci J, et al: Childhood bereavement: psychopathology in the 2 years postparental death. J Am Acad Child Adolesc Psychiatry 45(6):681–690, 2006 16721318

Claycomb MA, Charak R, Kaplow J, et al: Persistent Complex Bereavement Disorder symptom domains relate differentially to PTSD and depression: a study of war-exposed Bosnian adolescents. J Abnorm Child Psychol 44(7):1361–1373, 2016 26695010

Cohen JA, Mannarino AP: Treatment of childhood traumatic grief. J Clin Child Adolesc Psychol 33(4):819–831, 2004 15498749

Cohen JA, Mannarino AP, Greenberg T, et al: Childhood traumatic grief: concepts and controversies. Trauma Violence Abuse 3(4):307–437, 2002

Cohen JA, Mannarino AP, Staron VR: A pilot study of modified cognitive-behavioral therapy for childhood traumatic grief (CBT-CTG). J Am Acad Child Adolesc Psychiatry 45(12):1465–1473, 2006 17135992

Dowdney L: Annotation: childhood bereavement following parental death. J Child Psychol Psychiatry 41(7):819–830, 2003

Dowdney L, Wilson R, Maughan B, et al: Psychological disturbance and service provision in parentally bereaved children: prospective case-control study. BMJ 319(7206):354–357, 1999 10435957

Dyregrov K, Dyregrov A, Kristensen P: Traumatic bereavement and terror: the psychosocial impact on parents and siblings 1.5 years after the July 2011 terror killings in Norway. J Loss Trauma 20(6):556–576, 2015 21852658

Feigelman W, Rosen Z, Joiner T, et al: Examining longer-term effects of parental death in adolescents and young adults: evidence from the National Longitudinal Survey of Adolescent to Adult Health. Death Stud 41(3):133–143, 2017 27813715

Frederique N: What do the data reveal about violence in schools? Natl Inst Justice J 282:65–71, 2020

Giannopoulou I, Richardson C, Papadatou D: Peer loss: posttraumatic stress, depression, and grief symptoms in a traumatized adolescent community. Clin Child Psychol Psychiatry 26(2):556–568, 2021 33300387

Grenklo TB, Kreicbergs U, Hauksdóttir A, et al: Self-injury in teenagers who lost a parent to cancer: a nationwide, population-based, long-term follow-up. JAMA Pediatr 167(2):133–140, 2013

Hamdan S, Melhem NM, Porta G, et al: Alcohol and substance abuse in parentally bereaved youth. J Clin Psychiatry 74(8):828–833, 2013 24021502

Hill RM, Kaplow JB, Oosterhoff B, Layne CM: Understanding grief reactions, thwarted belongingness, and suicide ideation in bereaved adolescents: toward a unifying theory. J Clin Psychol 75(4):780–793, 2019 30636043

Hillis SD, Unwin HJT, Chen Y, et al: Global minimum estimates of children affected by COVID-19-associated orphanhood and deaths of caregivers: a modelling study. Lancet 398(10298):391–402, 2021

International Institute for Strategic Studies (ed): The IISS Armed Conflict Survey 2015: The Worldwide Review of Political, Military and Humanitarian Trends in Current Conflicts. London, Routledge, 2019

Kalantari M, Vostanis P: Behavioural and emotional problems in Iranian children four years after parental death in an earthquake. Int J Soc Psychiatry 56(2):158–167, 2010 20207678

Kaplow JB, Saunders J, Angold A, Costello EJ: Psychiatric symptoms in bereaved versus nonbereaved youth and young adults: a longitudinal epidemiological study. J Am Acad Child Adolesc Psychiatry 49(11):1145–1154, 2010 20970702

Kaplow JB, Layne CM, Pynoos RS, et al: DSM-V diagnostic criteria for bereavement-related disorders in children and adolescents: developmental considerations. Psychiatry 75(3):243–266, 2012 22913501

Kaplow JB, Layne CM, Oosterhoff B, et al: Validation of the Persistent Complex Bereavement Disorder (PCBD) Checklist: a developmentally informed assessment tool for bereaved youth. J Trauma Stress 31(2):244–254, 2018

Kentor RA, Kaplow JB: Supporting children and adolescents following parental bereavement: guidance for health-care professionals. Lancet Child Adolesc Health 4(12):889–898, 2020 33217358

Krause K: From armed conflict to political violence: mapping & explaining conflict trends. Daedalus 145(4):113–126, 2016

Kuramoto SJ, Stuart EA, Runeson B, et al: Maternal or paternal suicide and offspring's psychiatric and suicide-attempt hospitalization risk. Pediatrics 126(5):e1026–e1032, 2010

Layne CM, Saltzman WR, Poppleton L, et al: Effectiveness of a school-based group psychotherapy program for war-exposed adolescents: a randomized controlled trial. J Am Acad Child Adolesc Psychiatry 47(9):1048–1062, 2008 18664995

Li J, Vestergaard M, Cnattingius S, et al: Mortality after parental death in childhood: a nationwide cohort study from three Nordic countries. PLoS Med 11(7):e1001679, 2014 25051501

McKay MT, Cannon M, Healy C, et al: A meta-analysis of the relationship between parental death in childhood and subsequent psychiatric disorder. Acta Psychiatr Scand 143(6):472–486, 2021 33604893

Melhem NM, Day N, Shear MK, et al: Traumatic grief among adolescents exposed to a peer's suicide. Am J Psychiatry 161(8):1411–1416, 2004 15285967

Melhem NM, Moritz G, Walker M, et al: Phenomenology and correlates of complicated grief in children and adolescents. J Am Acad Child Adolesc Psychiatry 46(4):493–499, 2007 17420684

Melhem NM, Walker M, Moritz G, Brent DA: Antecedents and sequelae of sudden parental death in offspring and surviving caregivers. Arch Pediatr Adolesc Med 162(5):403–410, 2008 18458185

Melhem NM, Porta G, Shamseddeen W, et al: Grief in children and adolescents bereaved by sudden parental death. Arch Gen Psychiatry 68(9):911–919, 2011 21893658; erratum in JAMA Psychiatry 76:1319, 2019 21893658

Mie A: Orphans need special trauma care. The Japan Times, March 12, 2013. Available at: https://www.japantimes.co.jp/news/2013/03/12/national/orphans-need-special-trauma-care. Accessed December 1, 2021.

Nader KO: Childhood traumatic loss: The interaction of trauma and grief, in Death and Trauma: The Traumatology of Grieving. Edited by Figley CR, Bride BE, Mazza N. New York, Routledge, 1997, pp 17–41

Nicolson NA: Childhood parental loss and cortisol levels in adult men. Psychoneuroendocrinology 29(8):1012–1018, 2004 15219652

Normand CL, Silverman PR, Nickman SL: Bereaved children's changing relationships with the deceased, in Continuing Bonds: New Understanding of Grief. Edited by Klass D, Silverman PR, Nickman SL. Washington, DC, Taylor and Francis, 1996, pp 87–111

Oosterhoff B, Kaplow JB, Layne CM: Links between bereavement due to sudden death and academic functioning: results from a nationally representative sample of adolescents. Sch Psychol Q 33(3):372–380, 2018

Pham S, Porta G, Biernesser C, et al: The burden of bereavement: early-onset depression and impairment in youth bereaved by parental sudden death in a 7-year prospective study. Am J Psychiatry 175(9):887–896, 2018 29921145

Prigerson HG, Maciejewski PK, Reynolds CF III, et al: Inventory of complicated grief: a scale to measure maladaptive symptoms of loss. Psychiatry Res 59(1–2):65–79, 1995 8771222

Raveis VH, Siegel K, Karus D: Children's psychological distress following the death of a parent. J Youth Adolesc 28(2):165–180, 1999

Rotheram-Borus MJ, Murphy DA, Wight RG, et al: Improving the quality of life among young people living with HIV. Eval Program Plann 24(2):227–237, 2001

Rotheram-Borus MJ, Weiss R, Alber S, Lester P: Adolescent adjustment before and after HIV-related parental death. J Consult Clin Psychol 73(2):221–228, 2005 15796629

Sandler I, Ayers TS, Tein JY, et al: Six-year follow-up of a preventive intervention for parentally bereaved youths: a randomized controlled trial. Arch Pediatr Adolesc Med 164(10):907–914, 2010a 20921347

Sandler IN, Ma Y, Tein J-Y, et al: Long-term effects of the family bereavement program on multiple indicators of grief in parentally bereaved children and adolescents. J Consult Clin Psychol 78(2):131–143, 2010b 20350025

Sandler IN, Wolchik SA, Ayers TS, et al: Family Bereavement Program (FBP) approach to promoting resilience following the death of a parent. Fam Sci 4(1):87–94, 2013 24273631

Sandler I, Tein J-Y, Wolchik S, Ayers TS: The effects of the Family Bereavement Program to reduce suicide ideation and/or attempts of parentally bereaved children six and fifteen years later. Suicide Life Threat Behav 46(Suppl 1):S32–S38, 2016 27094109

Save the Children: State of the World's Mothers 2014: Saving Mothers and Children in Humanitarian Crises. Westport, CT, Save the Children, 2014

Servaty-Seib HL, Hayslip B Jr.: Post-loss adjustment and funeral perceptions of parentally bereaved adolescents and adults. Omega (Westport) 46(3):251–261, 2003

Slomski A: Thousands of US youths cope with the trauma of losing parents to COVID-19. JAMA 326(21):2117–2119, 2021 34787636

Spuij M, Prinzie P, Zijderlaan J, et al: Psychometric properties of the Dutch inventories of prolonged grief for children and adolescents. Clin Psychol Psychother 19(6):540–551, 2012 21774035

Stikkelbroek Y, Prinzie P, de Graaf R, et al: Parental death during childhood and psychopathology in adulthood. Psychiatry Res 198(3):516–520, 2012 22425472

Stikkelbroek Y, Bodden DHM, Reitz E, et al: Mental health of adolescents before and after the death of a parent or sibling. Eur Child Adolesc Psychiatry 25(1):49–59, 2016 25786705

Strøm IF, Schultz J-H, Wentzel-Larsen T, Dyb G: School performance after experiencing trauma: a longitudinal study of school functioning in survivors of the Utøya shootings in 2011. Eur J Psychotraumatol 7:31359, 2016 27171613

Thurman TR, Luckett BG, Nice J, et al: Effect of a bereavement support group on female adolescents' psychological health: a randomised controlled trial in South Africa. Lancet Glob Health 5(6):e604–e614, 2017 28462880

U.S. Census Bureau: Survey of income and program participation: 2014 panel wave 1. Unpublished raw data, 2014. Available at: https://census.gov/programs-surveys/sipp/data/datasets/2014-panel/wave-1.html. Accessed December 1, 2021.

Wardecker BM, Kaplow JB, Layne CM, Edelstein RS: Caregivers' positive emotional expression and children's psychological functioning after parental loss. J Child Fam Stud 26(12):3490–3501, 2017 29170615

Webb NB: Assessment of the bereaved child, in Helping Bereaved Children: A Handbook for Practitioners, 3rd Edition. Edited by Webb NB. New York, Guilford Press, 2010, pp 22–47

Weinberg RJ, Dietz LJ, Stoyak S, et al: A prospective study of parentally bereaved youth, caregiver depression, and body mass index. J Clin Psychiatry 74(8):834–840, 2013 24021503

Wilcox HC, Kuramoto SJ, Lichtenstein P, et al: Psychiatric morbidity, violent crime, and suicide among children and adolescents exposed to parental death. J Am Acad Child Adolesc Psychiatry 49(5):514–523, 2010 20431471

Yu Y, Liew Z, Cnattingius S, et al: Association of mortality with the death of a sibling in childhood. JAMA Pediatr 171(6):538–545, 2017 28437534

Clinical Management of Bereaved Patients With and Without Prolonged Grief Disorder

Alana Iglewicz, M.D.
Abigail Clark, M.D., Ph.D.
Sidney Zisook, M.D.

Whether or not we like to acknowledge it, death is always a part of life. In 2019, more than 2.8 million people died in the United States alone (Kochanek et al. 2020). The coronavirus pandemic added ~500,000 deaths in 2020, bringing the overall death rate well above 3 million. Each person who dies leaves behind an estimated nine close relatives and a number of other relatives and friends. This totals more than 27 million newly bereaved people in the United States in just one year (Verdery et al. 2020).

The vast majority of those who grieve can recover without needing professional help. However, a small but meaningful minority may struggle with persistent, impairing grief—a grief variant now called *prolonged grief disorder* (PGD) in both ICD-11 (World Health Organization 2022) and DSM-5-TR (American Psychiatric Association 2022)—and be vulnerable to other general medical and mental health conditions that sometimes arise or worsen in newly bereaved individuals. Individuals with PGD benefit from professional support (Shear et al. 2011, 2017; Zisook and Shear 2009; Zisook et al. 2014).

Based on the authors' extensive experience as both clinicians and clinical researchers on bereavement and PGD, in this chapter we describe an approach to assessment and compassionate, evidence-based bereavement care that can be provided in general medical and specialty mental health settings.

Clinical Management

Clinical management, which focuses on the patient rather than on the disease itself, refers to nonpharmacologic aspects of general medical or mental health care. Clinical management consists of a broad array of interventions and approaches:

- completing a thorough diagnostic assessment and treatment plan;
- establishing therapeutic rapport and maintaining an alliance with the patient;
- providing education to the patient and family;
- coordinating care with other clinicians;
- monitoring the patient's clinical status;
- integrating measurements into clinical management;
- enhancing treatment adherence; and
- assessing and attending to patient safety.

Ideally, clinicians provide these services throughout all phases of the patient's treatment.

Introducing Enhanced Clinical Management

One example of the clinical management of bereaved patients comes from a four-site study of the efficacy of antidepressant medication with or without grief-focused psychotherapy for PGD (called "complicated grief" in that study [Shear et al. 2016]). Participants randomly received one of four treatment conditions: antidepressant medication alone, placebo medication alone, antidepressant medication with complicated grief therapy (what is now termed *prolonged grief disorder therapy*, or PGDT), or placebo medication with PDGT. Patients in all four groups underwent *enhanced clinical management*, during which the clinicians

1. conducted an initial hour-long session to establish a therapeutic relationship and obtain a comprehensive history of the patient's relationship with the deceased;

2. acknowledged the importance of the patient's loss and the pain associated with such a loss;
3. provided hope through reassurance, information about the rationale, and a plan for treatment;
4. scheduled 20- to 30-minute follow-up sessions at regular intervals;
5. educated the patient about grief and PGD and encouraged them to ask questions and discuss concerns;
6. communicated with empathy and without judgment;
7. monitored grief, depression, side effects, and safety;
8. sought permission to speak with other providers and family as necessary; and
9. encouraged a healthy lifestyle, including attention to diet, exercise, socialization, and other activities.

In the study, antidepressant medication, as monotherapy or combined with PGDT, was not found to be efficacious; however, the study confirmed the robust efficacy of PGDT itself. The positive response rates were as follows: antidepressant alone, 69%; placebo alone, 55%; antidepressant + PGDT, 84%; and placebo + PGDT, 83%. Although grief-focused psychotherapy clearly was shown to be the treatment of choice, a notable finding was how well participants did who were assigned antidepressant/placebo without PGDT. This finding was especially striking considering that PGD tends to be chronic and debilitating without treatment—in fact, many of the study participants had lived with profound and persistent symptoms of PGD for years or even decades. The investigators attributed this surprising finding to the overall effectiveness of the one clinical approach received by all study participants: enhanced clinical management. Procedures for enhanced clinical management are delineated in the following sections, along with a discussion of how enhanced clinical management is applied during various periods of a patient's grief journey.

Assessment of Acute and Integrated Grief

Although there are questionnaires to measure acute grief (Faschingbauer et al. 1977) and screen for (Shear et al. 2006) or identify (Prigerson et al. 1995; 2021) PGD, clinical assessment is the preferred method to identify and understand acute and integrated grief. A few simple questions generally suffice: Has anyone close to you died? If so, how are you coping with your loss? Do you feel you have grieved? Are you adjusted to life without the person? Are you still struggling with your loss in any way? Do you feel frozen in your grief? Would it be OK if we talk about it?

Questions about important losses are a recommended part of a standard diagnostic evaluation. This is especially important with older patients, for whom loss is relatively common (Newson et al. 2011; Shear 2015). Risk factors that may alert clinicians to possible difficulties adapting to loss include multiple deaths and a history of mood, anxiety, or substance use disorders. Major depression early in bereavement increases the likelihood of PGD down the road (Guldin et al. 2017). Death of a child or a spouse, by any cause, is associated with heightened risk for PGD, as is loss of any loved one to suicide or other violent causes of death. Losing someone with whom one has had a close relationship can also be especially hard if the bereaved person had a difficult upbringing or if there are unusually stressful consequences of the death (i.e., inadequate social support, serious conflicts with friends or relatives, or major financial problems) (Shear 2015).

Clinicians are advised to be alert for any hints at recent or troublesome losses for all of their patients. When a patient shares that a loved one has died, one of the most valuable first steps is to recognize the import of the moment. Pause and allow the patient time to explain what happened. Set aside or curtail the original appointment agenda—be it medication follow-up, diagnostic evaluation, or completion of required annual screens. An expression of grief at any time should prompt clinicians to change what they are planning or doing to be fully present for the patient: for instance, to stop documenting in the medical record and shift full attention to the patient.

A one-time assessment is not enough. We recommend monitoring a bereaved individual over time until they have adapted to the loss and grief is diminished in overall intensity. Monitoring can be done with a few simple questions, such as: How are you coping with [name]'s death? How are you experiencing your grief? Is life without [name] becoming more bearable? How so? Clinicians can anticipate that most patients will adapt to loss by accepting the reality, consequences, and finality of the loss; altering their ongoing relationship with the deceased in a way that psychologically and spiritually works for them; and restoring their capacity for meaning and joy in life.

Management of Acute Grief

Typical, uncomplicated, acute grief is a normal, adaptive, and universal response to loss and should certainly not be pathologized. Yet all bereaved people benefit from compassionate support. Many turn to clinicians because they are discomfited by what they are experiencing and wonder if it is "normal." For many people, such as in the following case example, grief after losing someone very close is among the most intensely painful and disruptive experiences of their lives.

Case Example: Lila

Lila is a pleasant 70-year-old woman who has been a regular patient of yours for some time, but whom you have not seen for several months. Other than diuretics for hypertension, she is medication free. At a routine visit, you ask Lila about her family. She suddenly looks distraught and informs you that her husband of almost 40 years died 3 months ago from an unusual form of cancer. She goes on to tell you she cannot stop asking herself why he got cancer and why it couldn't be treated. She often thinks about why she did not figure out what was wrong before it was too late. Lila finds it difficult to look at pictures of her deceased husband or go to places that they used to go together, as both activities flood her with emotion. She questions her faith in God since her husband died. She skips meals because it is too hard to prepare them as she did for 45 years. She feels strangely incomplete with other people. She still has her job but often calls in sick. She sees her children regularly but does not feel as close to them anymore. She often finds herself daydreaming for hours about being with her husband. She has been so preoccupied with her grief that she sometimes misses taking her medications for hypertension. Friends and family, initially very supportive, tell her she needs to move on. Although Lila knows her husband would want her to be happy again, she does not see how it is possible after losing someone who was so much a part of her.

Clinicians can provide compassionate care for patients like Lila by accepting grief and bearing witness to the pain. An adage in medical education—"When you don't know what to do, just be human"—can help guide the approach to providing support.

Clinicians are advised to show natural human compassion for the loss, indicated with nonverbal as well as verbal communication. This means paying attention to tone of voice, use of pauses, and body language. Ideally, clinicians should use a kind, caring tone of voice. They should make a sympathetic statement about the loss (e.g.,"I am so sorry to hear that [name] died"), followed by a meaningful pause. Clinicians are encouraged to indicate through body language and other behavior that they are not hurried or distracted but rather prepared to be fully present and are interested in listening to the patient's story (Iglewicz et al. 2020; Shear et al. 2017). Table 3–1 provides several of the components of what we call enhanced clinical management for grief.

A desire to assuage grieving patients' pain and forge a connection may make clinicians tempted to offer platitudes, such as "at least he lived a long,

Table 3–1.   Grief-focused enhanced clinical management

Component	Example
Practice empathic, active listening	"I am so sorry for your loss. Please, tell me more."
Provide psychoeducation	"Grief is the form love takes when someone you love dies."
Name emotions	"I think what you are saying is how remorseful you are feeling; is that correct?"
Validate	"I can see how sad and empty you are feeling."
Normalize	"It is very common for people to carry on conversations with their deceased spouse. It is also really common for these grieving individuals to think they are going crazy when they have these conversations. Does that resonate with you?"
Monitor symptoms	"On a scale of 1 to 10, how intense has your grief been on most days since we last spoke? How frequent have the intense pangs been occurring? How long do they tend to last?"
Support a return to enjoyable activities without the deceased	"Do you feel ready go to your favorite restaurant? How about if your friend accompanies you? If not quite ready, how about just driving by for now?"
Treat co-occurring conditions	"In addition to working on your grief, how about if we begin to attend to your depression, which is also causing you pain?"
Offer guidance and resources	"Some patients have gotten a lot out of this [book/website/support group]. Would you consider attending a talk with others who have experienced [symptom]? Some people find the connection this offers to be very supportive and helpful."
Share judicious self-disclosure and lived experience	"I don't usually share my personal life with patients, but it might be useful to know that I also lost someone to [cause of death] and experienced [symptoms] for [duration]. I knew that nothing would ever be the same. Somehow, I eventually found…."
Refer for more focused PGD treatment as needed and available	"What you are going through is called *prolonged grief disorder*. There is a very effective type of psychotherapy for this condition. Would you be open to speaking with an expert on this treatment?"

full life" or "time heals all wounds," or to make claims that may be perceived by patients as insincere, such as "I understand." Remembering that grief is a form of love and therefore unique to each relationship, it is clear that no one really fully understands the nuances and complexity of thoughts and feelings engendered in someone else by the loss of a loved one. Thus, although well-intentioned, such comments are premised on false assumptions. They have the potential to miss the mark and make the patient feel more saddened, alone, and even angry (Iglewicz et al. 2020). Table 3–2 summarizes some of the recommended do's and don'ts of enhanced clinical management for grief-related support.

As a small, but powerful, touch, we recommend asking for the name of the loved one who died. It is warmer and more personal to use the person's name than to refer to "your husband," "your best friend," etc. (Iglewicz et al. 2020). We also recommend noting the name of the deceased loved one in the patient's medical chart, reviewing it before the next session, and using the name in subsequent visits. This small touch can speak volumes, humanizing the death and helping the patient feel more heard by and more connected with you.

Clinicians are encouraged to take the following approaches when interviewing patients about their grief experiences (Iglewicz et al. 2020):

- Invite the patient to talk about their relationship with the deceased, making no assumptions about the quality of that relationship;
- Create a safe environment in which the patient can disclose aspects of the relationship they cherished, as well as difficulties;
- Invite the patient to tell the story of the death, listening for how the person died; whether the death was expected, sudden, peaceful, or violent; and whether the patient was present at the death;
- Inquire what things have been like for the patient since the death, paying attention to grief symptoms and the effectiveness of available support;
- Ask who is available to support the patient and whether they have a close confidant with whom they can share painful thoughts and feelings, paying attention to whether there are friends, family, colleagues, or a religious community available for support.

If there is not time for this more comprehensive discussion, a shorter discussion about grief can still be a helpful start. In this shortened version, be sure to express genuine sympathy, find out the name of the loved one, and ask how the patient is coping with their grief. In addition, try to schedule a follow-up visit sooner than planned to talk more about their loss. Monitor the patient's progress in adapting to the loss at each visit until comfortable

Table 3–2.   Do's and don'ts

Do	Don't
Pause and listen	Keep typing
Ask for a name	Try to fix it
Inquire about the relationship and the grief	Make "at least" statements (such as "at least they died peacefully")
Be human	Use "should" statements
Assess for PGD and consider referral for PGDT where appropriate	Ask "why"
	Say you fully understand or that time heals all wounds

that they have successfully adapted. Look for evidence that the patient is both accepting the reality of this loss without protest and accepting the changed relationship with the person who died. In particular, look for a return of energy and enthusiasm for ongoing life and evidence that they have reengaged in ongoing, meaningful relationships.

In the case example, Lila's grief is intense and disabling but not particularly prolonged. She does not have PGD, but she is suffering. Upon learning of her loss, the clinician might first pause whatever else they are doing, put the computer to one side, lean forward, and express condolences: "I am so sorry for your loss" (pause). "This clearly has been quite painful for you" (pause). This might be followed by a comment such as "Can you remind me of your husband's name?" And then something like: "I missed out on getting to know John better, but the one thing I remember most is…." Time permitting, the clinician may ask more about how the two met, details of the relationship, how he died, and how she and the family are coping with and adapting to his death. Time not permitting, it is advisable to set up another appointment in the not-too-distant future to obtain this information and continue to offer support.

It is useful to listen nonjudgmentally and normalize grief symptoms: "Of course you are searching for what you could have done to save John and asking yourself 'Why?'" and "How could you not be grieving intensely for the man you have loved, lived with, and shared so much with for the majority of your life?" The clinician might follow such a comment with: "You loved him deeply. Grief is the form love takes when someone you love dies. The deeper the love, the more intense the grief can be." The therapist might even let Lila know that her well-meaning friends and family might not completely understand how deeply bereft she is. There is no simple fix. Her grief is natural, normal, acceptable, and probably even adaptive.

Before ending the session, the clinician will need to address Lila's self-care and medication adherence in a nonjudgmental and collaborative way: "Before we meet again next week, what can you and I do to get your blood pressure medications back on track?" At some point during this or the next session, it also is advisable to rule out major depression or other mental health problems, including thoughts of self-harm. The clinician does a complete review of symptoms, inquires about interpersonal and social supports, and asks Lila if there is anything else about John or her reaction to his death that they should talk about.

Management of Chronic Grief

Lila, *continued*

Three years later, Lila sees you again. It is now 39 months since John died, and her symptoms remain pronounced. Her loneliness is palpable. She is sad much of the time, but especially each night when she returns to an empty home. Every day, she is preoccupied with John's death, blaming herself for not catching his symptoms earlier; similarly, she remains angry at the doctors for not being able to cure John. Lila has not changed anything in the house since her husband died: his clothes and shoes are exactly where he left them. She avoids going to places they used to go together, including the supermarket and restaurants they used to frequent together. Additionally, she cannot bear to look at photographs of John. She often fantasizes about dying and joining him, and she often skips her hypertension medication, fully knowing this could be dangerous. Lila does not meet criteria for a major depressive episode and her general medical health is stable.

Grief is the natural response to the loss of a loved one. Hallmarks of acute grief include intense emotions, yearning, and preoccupation with thoughts and memories of the deceased person. Everyone grieves in their own way, and bereaved individuals often feel a sense of disconnection from themselves; from their past, present, and future; and especially from the person who died. They may fear never again being able to feel happy or fulfilled. Yet over time, most adapt to the loss, accepting its finality and consequences, including a changed relationship with the deceased, and reenvision a future with possibilities for happiness, joy, connection, and meaning—albeit in a world without the departed loved one.

A minority of bereaved patients will become caught up in ways of thinking, feeling, or acting that interfere with their ability to adapt to their loss (Shear et al. 2011; Zisook et al. 2014). As a result, acute grief symptoms may persist. Although there is no time frame for grief and no expectation that it is ever fully resolved, in most cultures and in most circumstances, the trajectory toward healing is well underway in 6–12 months. If that is not happening, the grief may be more accurately labeled *chronic* rather than *acute*. If the persistent grief also remains intense and disabling, it may be an instance of *prolonged grief disorder* (PGD), a serious condition that is associated with much suffering, mental and medical morbidity, and ongoing disability (Prigerson et al. 2021; Shear 2015; Shear et al. 2011).

The treatment principles described here apply to bereaved individuals regardless of time since the loved one's death, be it 3 months or 3 years. These approaches have direct applicability to grief support for patients both with and without PGD. Table 3–1 provides a concise list and several specific procedures for enhanced clinical management.

In the case example, Lila does not simply have chronic grief. She has PGD. Her grief is prolonged, intense, and disabling to a degree well beyond what is reasonably expected by anyone's cultural or religious norms. She may benefit from enhanced clinical management as outlined earlier, but PGDT (Shear 2015; Shear et al. 2016), if available, is the treatment of choice.

To treat PGD, several individual, group, and internet-based cognitive-behavioral treatments have been found to be effective in small randomized controlled trials (Boelen et al. 2007; Bryant et al. 2014; Kersting et al. 2013; Shear et al. 2005). A number of other authors have proposed various strategies and techniques for working with bereaved patients (Acierno et al. 2012; Asukai et al. 2011; Boelen et al. 2007; Neimeyer 2000; Rosner et al. 2011; Rynearson 1987; Wagner et al. 2006; Worden 2018). The most widely studied intervention, with by far the most evidence of efficacy, is prolonged grief disorder therapy. PGDT has been found to be robustly effective in three separate National Institute of Mental Health–sponsored randomized controlled trials, which included 641 adult patients who had lost a spouse, child, parent, sibling, or close friend by natural death or sudden violent death (Shear et al. 2005, 2014, 2016). As detailed in Chapter 7, PGDT helps promote adaptation to loss and restoration of life through seven healing milestones:

1. accepting grief;
2. managing emotions;
3. seeing a promising future;
4. strengthening relationships;
5. narrating a story of the death;
6. living with reminders; and
7. connecting with memories.

PGDT includes targeted procedures for each of these milestones, while keeping the therapy personalized and centered on active listening.

Applications in Diverse Clinical Settings

Time limitations and frequency of appointments vary in different practice settings. Clinicians also vary in their preferred way of working with patients. We suggest clinicians adapt the principles and procedures of enhanced clinical management and evidence-based grief therapy in the way that best fits their work. Next, we outline a possible approach for primary care physicians, pharmacotherapists, and psychotherapists.

Most bereaved patients, with or without PGD, benefit from any intervention that includes

- acknowledging their grief;
- bearing witness to their pain;
- being knowledgeable about grief and able to recognize PGD; and
- helping them to
  - tell the story of the death,
  - understand grief as a form of love,
  - learn to live in a world of reminders,
  - begin to envision and build an inviting future, and
  - maintain a comfortable awareness of their continuing relationship to the person who died.

When PGD is identified, a referral to PGDT or other evidence-based treatment is strongly encouraged. Alternatively, integration of the seven themes of PGDT into the clinical setting is recommended. A detailed discussion of how this might be done is provided in Chapter 7. A "bare bones" version includes

1. acknowledging the loss and expressing condolences;
2. empathically eliciting the narrative of the patient's relationship with the deceased loved one and the death;
3. discussing the PGD diagnosis with the patient;
4. providing grief-focused clinical management and, ideally, referral to specialty care; and
5. regularly checking in regarding the grief experience until the patient is able to accept the reality of the loss and restore their capacity for well-being.

The clinician does not expect to eliminate grief, but rather to help a patient accept grief as a part of learning to adapt to the loss while retaining the capacity for engaging in a life with possibilities for meaning and happiness.

For primary care physicians, this "bare bones" approach consists of acknowledging, listening, educating, referring, and monitoring. For psychiatrists whose practices are primarily focused on medication management, a referral to PGDT is the first-line approach. Alternatively, an enhanced intervention as described previously or in Chapter 7 might be considered. Principles of clinical management described in this chapter can be transported into the "20-minute hour." However, it is ideal to see the patient more frequently than may be customary in most practices, especially for the first few months after the loss. For psychotherapists (including psychiatrists who focus their practice on psychotherapy) who typically spend more time with patients at more frequent intervals, clinical management can be integrated into usual care. However, we strongly recommend that psychotherapists learn about PGD and its evidence-based treatments. For those clinicians who are interested in working with bereaved individuals, a variety of training opportunities are available to learn PGDT as detailed in Chapter 7. For example, in training provided by the Center for Prolonged Grief (Columbia University School of Social Work, New York), clinicians are encouraged to use principles, strategies, and procedures in their own way and to monitor outcomes.

Grief After Suicide

When a person loses a loved one to suicide, they often face unique challenges that differ markedly from the challenges after other types of death. In addition to the typical grief, sadness, and disbelief, proximity to suicide often brings overwhelming guilt, confusion, rejection, shame, and anger. These painful experiences may be further complicated by the effects of stigma and trauma. It is no surprise that those bereaved by suicide report higher incidences of rejection, blaming, shame, stigma, and the need to conceal the cause of death (compared with those bereaved by other causes of death). These themes are illustrated in the following case example.

Case Example: Sheila

Bill, a 51-year-old married man with two children, died by suicide 1½ years ago, a self-inflicted gunshot wound to the head. The first to find him was his wife, Sheila. He was in their car, which was parked in their garage, with a bag over his head, presumably placed to limit the "mess" of his gunshot. Sheila was shocked by her husband's suicide and has been consumed by grief ever since.

In her mind, Sheila replays the days that led up to his death, combing them for any and all possibilities of preventing it. She is consumed by the "what ifs, could haves, and should haves." She second-guesses herself: "if only I had said something," "if only I did not go to work that day," "I should have recognized the signs," "I could have stopped this from happening." She is filled with anger—toward him, toward herself, and toward his boss. She wonders, "Why would he do this?," "Why didn't his boss give him the promotion he so deserved?," "How could he leave our children behind?," "How could he have left me alone?," "Did he not love us enough?" Her anger is intertwined with guilt. In addition to guilt about not preventing his suicide, she experiences guilt about feeling anger. Whenever she recognizes that he must have been suffering terribly to choose to end his life, she then berates herself for being angry at him for his death.

Sheila is simultaneously burdened by profound sadness. Her sadness comes in waves. She has near-daily crying spells. Reminders of Bill, such as smelling his cologne or hearing a favorite song of his on the radio, induce sobbing. She avoids going to places they used to enjoy together and avoids spending time with their mutual friends and family—the memories these places and people evoke are too painful. She avoids removing any of Bill's possessions. His possessions remain where he left them. Every day, she lies in bed crying, while hugging and smelling a sweatshirt he left on their bed before his death. It remains unwashed. She feels overwhelmed with parenting responsibilities and financial matters. Bill had been in charge of their finances, and she questions how she can manage without him—both literally and figuratively. When Sheila feels particularly overwhelmed, she has fleeting thoughts of "joining Bill." She vows not to act on these thoughts, as she knows the pain of losing a loved one to suicide and does not want to be the cause of added suffering for her children.

Not a day has passed since his death that Sheila does not think of the image of Bill's bloodied, unrecognizable face inside the plastic bag. The image haunts her. She sees it in her waking hours, and the image even wakes her from sleep. Despite the significant impairment she experiences, she has not sought help. She fears that talking about her husband's death and her grief will only make it worse. She also avoids talking with family and friends about the profundity of her grief. She senses they are uncomfortable with her pain and emotionality and also that Bill died by suicide. Sheila is embarrassed to tell people how her husband died, feeling ashamed by her inability to have prevented the death of the man she loved since the day they met 30 years ago. Since his death, her grief surges on the date of his birthday, their wedding anniversary, their children's birthdays, and the holidays. Her grief was especially heightened surrounding the 1-year anniversary of Bill's death.

Although everyone experiences grief in their own unique way, this case example highlights some of the main themes emblematic of suicide bereavement: the context of stigma, preoccupying themes, and commonly associated comorbidities.

Stigma Related to Suicide Loss

One of the major contributors to the complexity and pain of suicide bereavement is the associated stigma (Jordan 2008; Tal et al. 2017; Tal Young et al. 2012). Despite impressive efforts by many organizations aimed at decreasing the stigma of mental illness, and more specifically suicide, the stigma shrouding suicide remains pervasive. We see it in insurance policies, certain religious beliefs and practices, and until relatively recently, the practices of the U.S. military. (It was not until 2011 that our government began honorably acknowledging military families bereaved by suicide with the presidential condolence letters similar to those sent to families bereaved by deaths occurring in combat [Cozza et al. 2019].)

Family members and friends often do not know how to best support those bereaved by suicide. They feel awkward and helpless and end up avoiding interactions with the person mourning, who internalizes these layers of stigma. The resulting shame leads many to conceal the cause of death and avoid discussing the suicide to prevent themselves and others from feeling uncomfortable. Isolation and loneliness ensue. As we saw with Sheila, the suicide bereaved are then deprived of the very sources of support that are key to healing after any loss—and that are essential after a loss as devastating as suicide.

Common Themes

We are faced with a challenging paradox in our field. From a mental health professional and public health standpoint, we need to do everything possible to prevent suicides. We thus have numerous campaigns aimed at this important goal. From a grief standpoint, the belief that suicide is preventable leads to a dangerous cascade of thoughts and feelings that complicate the grief experience. The bereaved typically believe that suicide is preventable and that it reflects a poor decision on the part of the person who died by suicide. These perceptions set the stage for displaced and projected anger, feelings of abandonment, and ruminating self-doubt (Shear and Zisook 2014). As with Sheila, the bereaved are consumed by "what ifs." They dwell on the days before the suicide, trying to convince themselves that if only they had done or said something different, their loved one would still be alive (Tal Young et al. 2012). Because marriage is typically the most intimate relationship people have, individuals such as Sheila whose spouses die by suicide are often consumed by feelings of rejection and abandonment. They question why they weren't enough for their loved one to choose life over death (Cerel et al. 2008).

Another common theme of suicide bereavement is anger. As with Sheila, common foci of the anger include oneself for not preventing the suicide; the deceased for choosing suicide; colleagues or others for possible contributions to the suicide; and caregivers, friends, family members, health care providers, and religious figures such as God. At times the anger is pervasive and mixed with envy. It becomes directed toward the world and all the people who have never experienced the pain of suicide loss (Tal Young et al. 2012).

Comorbidities

Considering that suicide is inherently violent, traumatic, and unnatural, and considering the stigma, shame, anger, rejection, confusion, and guilt associated with suicide loss, those bereaved by suicide are at increased risk for various psychiatric comorbidities. These include major depressive disorder (MDD), PTSD, suicidal ideation and behaviors, and PGD (see Chapter 5). In light of her crying spells, isolation, guilt, and suicidal ideation, Sheila should be carefully assessed for MDD, and considering the intrusive images of her husband's face after his death, PTSD should also be on the differential. Additionally, she has many symptoms of PGD. These include avoidance (evading reminders of her husband), as well as the converse, proximity-seeking (keeping his belongings untouched and holding his unwashed sweatshirt), anger, yearning, and suicidal thoughts. When a patient has symptoms and is impaired, PGD may be diagnosed 12 months after the loved one's death (6 months for children and adolescents). However, suicide bereavement tends to persist longer than traditional grief (Feigelman et al. 2009). (This leads to questions about the applicability of the PGD criteria to the timeline for "normal" grief after suicide.) All that being said, we know that PGD symptoms may persist indefinitely when untreated, leaving the bereaved frozen in the pronounced acute stages of their grief, with significant associated morbidity and even mortality. In contrast, when properly managed, PGD has an excellent prognosis (Shear et al. 2016).

Treatment Considerations

If a patient has suspected psychiatric comorbidities, the key is to assess for and then optimally treat them. One should think in terms of *and* rather than *or*. Rather than ask whether this is grief or MDD, for example, ask whether it is grief *and* the other condition. When a comorbid mental health condition is present, it is essential to provide compassionate, thoughtful, efficacious treatment for that condition while simultaneously addressing the grief.

Of course, not everyone who is grieving the loss of a loved one to suicide has psychiatric comorbidities. Grief is a natural, adaptive process that should not be pathologized or medicalized. In addition, there is no doubt that grieving the loss of a loved one to suicide has layers of complexity. Whether or not comorbidities are present, focused support groups can be very helpful. Support groups focused on suicide bereavement are a safe haven in which participants learn from others who have done—and have supported others in doing—the unimaginable feat of devising and enacting new goals for a life that will forever be marked by this immense, inconceivable loss. By participating in a support group, Sheila can lessen the shame, stigma, and isolation she feels. With evaluation and treatment for MDD, trauma, and PGD, she can slowly and rightfully regain her life. The positive sequelae of her treatment can be profound, adding meaning and connection to her relationships with her children, other family members, and friends, thus decreasing the risk for future suicide in her family for generations to come. Without that treatment and support, the results for herself and her loved ones can be devastating.

When a Clinician Loses a Patient to Suicide

Losing a patient to suicide is an occupational hazard for clinicians who treat patients with chronic and severe mental illnesses. At least half of psychiatrists and ~20% of psychologists, clinical social workers, and other mental health professionals will lose a patient to suicide in the course of their careers (Gutin 2019). Residents early in their training and other novice clinicians experience even higher rates of patient suicide than more seasoned clinicians.

Clinicians are human. They are not immune to grief after the death of people close to them, including their patients, especially those who die by suicide while entrusted to their care. The death of a patient by suicide is psychologically traumatic; it may even be a career-ending event. In the aftermath of a patient suicide, mental health professionals often blame themselves about self-perceived omissions or commissions. Driven by shame, fear, and stigma, they often will not discuss these events with colleagues, friends, or supervisors, let alone schedule therapy with a fellow professional.

Unlike most other physicians in medicine, psychiatrists do not often conceptualize the illnesses they treat as being potentially fatal or terminal. But they are. About 90% of individuals who die by suicide have mental illness. Mood disorders are among the most robust risk factors for suicide. Yet mental health professionals tend to rely on certain myths that interfere with their ability to accept patient suicide as a consequence of the patient's mental illness and life circumstances, rather than the clinician's failure.

One such myth is that effective clinical care can prevent all suicides. Clinicians can assess risk factors and do what they can to address the reversible ones (e.g., have a safety plan, reduce access to means, and treat comorbid conditions), but minimizing risk is not the same thing as preventing suicide. Not all suicides can be prevented, even by the most skilled and experienced clinicians. Suicide risk is complex and determined by multiple factors, including potentially lethal or malignant psychiatric conditions and traumatic life events that may occur between sessions (Moutier et al. 2021b).

A second prevalent myth is that with properly formed attachments and rapport in treatment, a patient would not "do that to me." Strong rapport is indeed a protective factor, but other risk factors operate outside the therapeutic setting. Love is not always enough. Empathy is imperfect. The acute suffering and cognitive constriction during a suicide storm sometimes override the protective effect of compassionate care.

A third myth is that truly skilled and compassionate clinicians can predict suicide and thus prevent it. But even the most skilled clinicians lose patients to suicide. More than half of suicides are by people who are not considered high risk, and an abundance of evidence demonstrates our inability to accurately predict suicide (Franklin et al. 2017). Again, risk and prediction are not the same.

In many ways, clinicians' responses after a patient's suicide are similar to those of other survivors of a loved one lost to suicide. Responses include rumination over myriad "why" questions; feelings of guilt, shame, and self-doubt; and a heightened sense of one's responsibility for the death—all magnified by the mythology noted previously and the stigma surrounding suicide. Table 3–3 lists some typical reactions clinicians experience after a patient suicide.

The shame clinicians often feel is a product of our tendency to overestimate our power. Mental health clinicians sometimes feel they can outwrestle death itself. When a patient dies by suicide, clinicians may have a sense of personal failure, self-doubt, guilt, and shame. Consequently, they may be tempted to hide their shame and withdraw from the help and support of others. They may feel like impostors, believe they are in the wrong field, and consider a change of profession or premature retirement. Their behavior with other patients may be altered, leading to hypervigilance and a tendency to overmedicate, overhospitalize, or avoid treating high-risk patients. They may overpersonalize, believing the patient did this specifically to them, and consequently feel rejected or abandoned. Relief that the patient is no longer suffering or no longer their responsibility may be tinged with guilt for feeling that way.

Table 3–3.   Clinician reactions to a patient death by suicide

Reaction	Example
Shame	"I didn't see this coming." "I am not clinically skilled."
Shaken confidence, doubt	"Maybe I am in the wrong career." "I failed."
Hypervigilance or avoidance	"I better hospitalize anyone with suicidal thoughts." "I shouldn't take on any patients with serious mental illness."
Guilt	"Should have" and "What if"
Rejection, abandonment	"They left me." "Why was my care for this patient not enough?"
Anger	"How could they do this to me?"
Relief	"At least I can stop worrying."
Other stress, trauma, and loss symptoms	"I can't sleep."

For clinicians to adapt to the suicide of a patient and mitigate the potential adverse outcomes, the first step is preventive: comprehensive education on suicide prevention during both career training and continuing education. Such education should include learning to identify risk factors and warning signs, apply safety plans and evidence-based interventions, and make realistic appraisals of prediction and prevention. We recommend that psychiatry residency programs provide suicide education early in training and pair it with firsthand testimonies of patients who have survived suicide attempts and residents and faculty who have had patients die by suicide—sessions that ensure opportunities for discussion. These approaches help provide trainees with the best available information, competence, and foreknowledge that patient suicides are tragic but not always preventable.

Trainees should be taught that they are not alone if a patient dies by suicide. The video "Collateral Damages: The Impact of Patient Suicide on the Physician" features several physicians speaking about their experiences losing a patient to suicide, as well as a group discussion (Prabhakar et al. 2013, 2014). This resource can be used to facilitate an educational session for physicians, psychologists, residents, and other trainees. It is available for educational use by contacting education@afsp.org and for psychiatry residency training programs through the American Association for Directors of Psychiatry Residency Training (AADPRT) website. Several other curricula for helping residents cope with patient suicide have been proposed (Lerner et al. 2012; Lomax 1986; McCutcheon and Hyman 2021; Whitmore et al. 2017). What these curricula have in common is recognizing the importance of breaking through the shroud of silence surrounding patient suicide, using strategies to destigmatize and universalize the experience, providing support and a sense of community, and disseminating relevant information, resources, and processes to follow.

Next, in each academic setting or institution, there should be a plan for how support is provided when a patient dies by suicide. Several institutional guidelines are available (Dyrbye et al. 2017, 2018; Quinnett 1999; Sung 2016). These include recommendations for providing information in the most sensitive way possible to those who need to know and discussions of legal and ethical issues. Guidelines also suggest that suicide postvention policies and protocols be in place from the outset, and that such information be incorporated into institutional policy and procedure manuals.

Guidelines for individual clinicians who experience a patient's suicide also are available (Grad 2009; Gutin 2018; Quinnett 1999; Sung 2016). These guidelines notably share an emphasis on talking about the loss and connecting with others. Sharing these experiences in a supportive atmosphere helps clinicians become more aware and accepting of their own therapeutic limitations, view their grief with self-compassion, and use this knowledge to better determine how they will continue their clinical work (Gutin 2019). Trainees and clinicians also need to be educated on the importance of timely documentation; the roles of legal representation and risk management; the limits of patient confidentiality; if, when, and how to contact the family; the pros and cons of attending the funeral; and opportunities for posttrauma growth (Gutin 2019). Not infrequently, clinicians receive conflicting advice on issues such as how open to be with surviving family or whether to attend funerals. While detailed discussions of these issues are beyond the scope of this chapter, we recommend, above all else, to be human and do what your heart and soul tells you is the right thing. When in doubt, obtaining and documenting a consultation with a colleague or supervisor can be useful.

Clinician and Personal Suicide Loss

Patient death by suicide is not a clinician's only exposure to suicide. Suicide on the part of physicians and other mental health professionals is common and is starting to receive much-needed attention. Each year, about 400 physicians die by suicide in the United States alone. Indeed, suicide is the leading cause of death among male residents and the second leading cause among female residents (Yaghmour et al. 2017). The risk likely increases throughout one's career, especially for women (Duarte et al. 2020; Dutheil et al. 2019; Ye et al. 2020). Additionally, both male and female nurses have higher rates of suicide than age-matched men and women in the general population (Davidson et al. 2020). As with all suicides, the impact of each loss extends beyond family and friends to peers, classmates, deans, institutional officials, and patients, and the psychological reactions include shock, anxiety, sorrow, guilt, self-blame, and fear. Because suicide is a complex health outcome with many drivers of risk, preventing suicide among health care workers requires a strategic, multipronged, longitudinal, evidence-based plan. Reducing the risk of clinician suicide requires changes in regulatory policies, changes in curricula, role modeling in medical education, increased access to mental health care, and transformation of an entrenched culture (Moutier et al. 2021a).

Most of us know someone who has died by suicide. These are inevitably tragic losses, leaving the bereaved with more questions than answers. In the circumstances, these deaths and subsequent grief can remind us to be kinder, humbler, more thoughtful, more caring, and more present human beings.

Teaching ourselves, our colleagues, and the public about how to optimally support those who are grieving the loss of a loved one to suicide is an important step in preventing suicide. If suicide bereavement can have intergenerational effects, so too can the interventions. Moreover, understanding loss allows us to understand and engage in life. For it is when we truly understand the pain of loss that we are inspired to address this important matter: to do what we can to empathically support those who are grieving, to provide optimal care to those at risk for suicide, and to advocate for policy change to address stigma, suicide prevention, and barriers to mental health care (Moutier et al. 2021a).

Prevention of PGD

While we have effective treatments for PGD once it develops, far less is known about preventing the development of PGD. One approach may be to attend to known, reversible risk factors, such as depression, anxiety, or substance use disorders. A few innovative studies have pointed to the potential role of enhanced end-of-life care in protecting against the later development of grief-related problems in the bereaved.

In the first of these, Wright et al. (2008) suggested a possible step to reduce bereavement-related distress in caregivers: reducing aggressive end-of-life medical care. In the study, aggressive medical care included ICU admission, ventilation, resuscitation, chemotherapy, or use of a feeding tube near death. More aggressive medical care was associated not only with worse quality of life in terminally ill patients but also with worse bereavement adjustment in caregivers, including increased rates of MDD, as measured 6.5 months later.

Place of death also appears to be an important factor affecting caregiver bereavement (Wright et al. 2010). Dying in a hospital or ICU was found to be associated with worse quality of life for terminally ill cancer patients compared with dying at home, and importantly, place of death mattered for outcomes of the bereaved caregivers as well. Caregivers of patients who died in a hospital were at increased risk for developing PGD, and caregivers of patients who died in the ICU were at increased risk for developing PTSD, compared with caregivers of patients who died at home with hospice care. These findings suggest that hospice interventions improve not only quality of life for terminally ill patients but also bereavement adjustment in their caregivers. Hospice care may therefore be an important component of preventing PGD.

In a third study, Garrido and Prigerson (2014) found several additional factors that predicted improved adjustment for bereaved caregivers, such as better quality of death; completion of a DNR order; and, in the caregivers themselves, better mental health and less pain before the loss. A more recent study (Falzarano et al. 2021) confirmed that completion of a DNR order in terminally ill cancer patients leads to decreased levels of grief in caregivers following the loss.

These findings reinforce the role of hospice care and advanced care planning in end-of-life settings. They indicate several possible areas of intervention and point toward hospice care being an important component of care for both the patient and the caregiver. Additional research is needed to determine targets of intervention for bereavement adjustment in relationships outside of the caregiver role and modes of death not limited to terminal illnesses but also including suicide. For unexpected or sudden death, targets of intervention before the death may not be possible, so it is important to also examine novel post-death interventions for the caregiver, such as individual or group therapy, a modified version of PGDT or other grief-specific therapy for high-risk groups, and even innovative pharmacologic approaches (Dos Santos et al. 2021).

Conclusion

Grief is a natural, instinctive, and adaptive process that typically warrants not treatment, but rather support. The one form of grief that requires treatment is prolonged grief disorder. This chapter on enhanced clinical management delineates a compassionate approach to grief in all of its forms—whether it be acute, integrated, or prolonged. Variations on this approach for different clinical settings are reviewed, as are special circumstances that add nuance to the support needs of the bereaved. The latter include individuals grieving the death of a loved one by suicide and clinicians grieving patients who die by suicide—both of whom face unique challenges and thematic content related to the stigma shrouding this type of death. Because preventing PGD in the first place is ideal, the extant literature on PGD prevention, including the role of hospice care and DNR orders in the terminally ill, is highlighted. Learning the enhanced clinical management of grief helps clinicians have more comfort, agility, and sophistication in their support of bereaved patients.

References

Acierno R, Rheingold A, Amstadter A, et al: Behavioral activation and therapeutic exposure for bereavement in older adults. Am J Hosp Palliat Care 29(1):13–25, 2012 21685428

American Psychiatric Association: Diagnostic and Statistical Manual of Mental Disorders, 5th Edition, Text Revision. Washington, DC, American Psychiatric Association, 2022

Asukai N, Tsuruta N, Saito A: Pilot study on traumatic grief treatment program for Japanese women bereaved by violent death. J Trauma Stress 24(4):470–473, 2011 21780192

Boelen PA, de Keijser J, van den Hout MA, van den Bout J: Treatment of complicated grief: a comparison between cognitive-behavioral therapy and supportive counseling. J Consult Clin Psychol 75(2):277–284, 2007

Bryant RA, Kenny L, Joscelyne A, et al: Treating prolonged grief disorder: a randomized clinical trial. JAMA Psychiatry 71(12):1332–1339, 2014 25338187

Cerel J, Jordan JR, Duberstein PR: The impact of suicide on the family. Crisis 29(1):38–44, 2008 18389644

Cozza S, Harrington-LaMorie J, Fisher JE: US military service deaths: Bereavement in surviving families, in American Military Life in the 21st Century: Social, Cultural and Economic Issues and Trends. Santa Barbara, CA, ABC-CLIO, 2019, pp 411–425

Davidson JE, Proudfoot J, Lee K, et al: A longitudinal analysis of nurse suicide in the United States (2005–2016) with recommendations for action. Worldviews Evid Based Nurs 17(1):6–15, 2020 32017434

Dos Santos RG, Bouso JC, Rocha JM, et al: The use of classic hallucinogens/psychedelics in a therapeutic context: healthcare policy opportunities and challenges. Risk Manag Healthc Policy 14:901–910, 2021

Duarte D, El-Hagrassy MM, Couto TCE, et al: Male and female physician suicidality: a systematic review and meta-analysis. JAMA Psychiatry 77(6):587–597, 2020 32129813

Dutheil F, Aubert C, Pereira B, et al: Suicide among physicians and health-care workers: a systematic review and meta-analysis. PLoS One 14(12):e0226361, 2019 31830138

Dyrbye L, Konopasek L, Moutier C: After a Suicide: A Toolkit for Physician Residency/Fellowship Programs. American Foundation for Suicide Prevention (AFSP) and the Mayo Clinic, 2017. Available at: http://www.acgme.org/Portals/0/PDFs/13287_AFSP_After_Suicide_Clinician_Toolkit_Final_2.pdf. Accessed March 23, 2023.

Dyrbye L, Moutier C, Wolanskyj-Spinner A, Zisook S: After a Suicide: A Toolkit for Medical Schools. New York, American Foundation for Suicide Prevention, 2018. Available at: https://www.afsp.org/physician. Accessed March 23, 2023.

Falzarano F, Prigerson HG, Maciejewski PK: The role of advance care planning in cancer patient, caregiver grief resolution: helpful or harmful? Cancers (Basel) 13(8):1977, 2021 33924214

Faschingbauer TR, Devaul RA, Zisook S: Development of the Texas Inventory of Grief. Am J Psychiatry 134(6):696–698, 1977

Feigelman W, Jordan JR, Gorman BS: How they died, time since loss, and bereavement outcomes. Omega 58:251–273, 2009

Franklin JC, Ribeiro JD, Fox KR, et al: Risk factors for suicidal thoughts and behaviors: a meta-analysis of 50 years of research. Psychol Bull 143(2):187–232, 2017 27841450

Garrido MM, Prigerson HG: The end-of-life experience: modifiable predictors of caregivers' bereavement adjustment. Cancer 120(6):918–925, 2014 24301644

Grad OT: Therapists as survivors of suicide loss, in Oxford Textbook of Suicidology and Suicide Prevention. Edited by Wasserman D, Wasserman C. Oxford, UK, Oxford Academic, 2009, pp 609–615

Guldin M-B, Kjaersgaard MIS, Fenger-Grøn M, et al: Risk of suicide, deliberate self-harm and psychiatric illness after the loss of a close relative: a nationwide cohort study. World Psychiatry 16(2):193–199, 2017 28498584

Gutin NJ: Helping survivors in the aftermath of suicide loss. Curr Psychiatry 17(8):27–33, 2018

Gutin NJ: Losing a patient to suicide: navigating the aftermath. Curr Psychiatry 18(11):17–24, 2019

Iglewicz A, Shear MK, Reynolds CF III, et al: Complicated grief therapy for clinicians: an evidence-based protocol for mental health practice. Depress Anxiety 37(1):90–98, 2020 31622522

Jordan JR: Bereavement after suicide. Psychiatr Ann 38(10):679–685, 2008

Kersting A, Dölemeyer R, Steinig J, et al: Brief internet-based intervention reduces post-traumatic stress and prolonged grief in parents after the loss of a child during pregnancy: a randomized controlled trial. Psychother Psychosomat 82(6):372–381, 2013

Kochanek KD, Xu J, Arias E: Mortality in the United States, 2019. NCHS Data Brief No. 395. Hyattsville, MD, National Center for Health Statistics, 2020

Lerner U, Brooks K, McNiel DE, et al: Coping with a patient's suicide: a curriculum for psychiatry residency training programs. Acad Psychiatry 36(1):29–33, 2012 22362433

Lomax JW: A proposed curriculum on suicide care for psychiatry residency. Suicide Life Threat Behav 16(1):56–64, 1986 3961882

McCutcheon S, Hyman J: Increasing resident support following patient suicide: assessing resident perceptions of a longitudinal, multimodal patient suicide curriculum. Acad Psychiatry 45(3):288–291, 2021 33655455

Moutier CY, Myers MF, Feist JB, et al: Preventing clinician suicide: a call to action during the COVID-19 pandemic and beyond. Acad Med 96(5):624–628, 2021a

Moutier C, Stahl SM, Pisani AR: Suicide Prevention: Stahl's Handbooks. Cambridge, UK, Cambridge University Press, 2021b

Neimeyer RA: Searching for the meaning of meaning: grief therapy and the process of reconstruction. Death Stud 24(6):541–558, 2000

Newson RS, Boelen PA, Hek K, et al: The prevalence and characteristics of complicated grief in older adults. J Affect Disord 132(1–2):231–238, 2011 21397336

Prabhakar D, Anzia JM, Balon R, et al: "Collateral damages": preparing residents for coping with patient suicide. Acad Psychiatry 37(6):429–430, 2013

Prabhakar D, Balon R, Anzia JM, et al: Helping psychiatry residents cope with patient suicide. Acad Psychiatry 38(5):593–597, 2014

Prigerson HG, Maciejewski PK, Reynolds CF III, et al: Inventory of Complicated Grief: a scale to measure maladaptive symptoms of loss. Psychiatry Res 59(1–2):65–79, 1995 8771222

Prigerson HG, Boelen PA, Xu J, et al: Validation of the new DSM-5-TR criteria for prolonged grief disorder and the PG-13-Revised (PG-13-R) scale. World Psychiatry 20(1):96–106, 2021 33432758

Quinnett P: QPR Institute Administrative Directory. Spokane, WA, QPR Institute, 1999 26640420

Rosner R, Pfoh G, Kotoucova M: Treatment of complicated grief. Eur J Psychotraumatol 2:7995, 2011 22893810

Rynearson EK: Psychotherapy of pathologic grief: revisions and limitations. Psychiatr Clin North Am 10(3):487–499, 1987 3684750

Shear MK: Clinical practice: complicated grief. N Engl J Med 372(2):153–160, 2015 25564898

Shear MK, Zisook S: Suicide-related bereavement and grief, in A Concise Guide to Understanding Suicide: Epidemiology, Pathophysiology and Prevention. Edited by Koslow SH, Ruiz P, Nemeroff CB. Cambridge, UK, Cambridge University Press, 2014, pp. 66–73 11532739

Shear K, Frank E, Houck PR, Reynolds CF III: Treatment of complicated grief: a randomized controlled trial. JAMA 293(21):2601–2608, 2005 15928281

Shear KM, Jackson CT, Essock SM, et al: Screening for complicated grief among Project Liberty service recipients 18 months after September 11, 2001. Psychiatr Serv 57(9):1291–1297, 2006 16968758

Shear MK, Simon N, Wall M, et al: Complicated grief and related bereavement issues for DSM-5. Depress Anxiety 28(2):103–117, 2011 21284063

Shear MK, Wang Y, Skritskaya N, et al: Treatment of complicated grief in elderly persons: a randomized clinical trial. JAMA Psychiatry 71(11):1287–1295, 2014 25250737

Shear MK, Reynolds CF III, Simon NM, et al: Optimizing treatment of complicated grief: a randomized clinical trial. JAMA Psychiatry 73(7):685–694, 2016 27276373

Shear MK, Muldberg S, Periyakoil V: Supporting patients who are bereaved. BMJ 358:j2854, 2017

Sung JC: Sample Agency Practices for Responding to Client Suicide. Oklahoma City, OK, Suicide Prevention Resource Center, 2016. Available at: https://sprc.org/sites/default/files/resource-program/Sample_Agency_Practices.pdf. Accessed March 23, 2023.

Tal I, Mauro C, Reynolds CF III, et al: Complicated grief after suicide bereavement and other causes of death. Death Stud 41(5):267–275, 2017 27892842

Tal Young I, Iglewicz A, Glorioso D, et al: Suicide bereavement and complicated grief. Dialogues Clin Neurosci 14(2):177–186, 2012 22754290

Verdery AM, Smith-Greenaway E, Margolis R, Daw J: Tracking the reach of COVID-19 kin loss with a bereavement multiplier applied to the United States. Proc Natl Acad Sci USA 117(30):17695–17701, 2020 32651279

Wagner B, Knaevelsrud C, Maercker A: Internet-based cognitive-behavioral therapy for complicated grief: a randomized controlled trial. Death Stud 30(5):429–453, 2006 16610157

Whitmore CA, Cook J, Salg L: Supporting residents in the wake of patient suicide. Am J Psychiatry Resid J 12(1):5–7, 2017

Worden JW: Grief Counseling and Grief Therapy, 5th Edition: A Handbook for the Mental Health Practitioner. New York, Springer, 2018

World Health Organization: International Statistical Classification of Diseases and Related Health Problems, 11th Revision. Geneva, World Health Organization, 2022

Wright AA, Zhang B, Ray A, et al: Associations between end-of-life discussions, patient mental health, medical care near death, and caregiver bereavement adjustment. JAMA 300(14):1665–1673, 2008 18840840

Wright AA, Keating NL, Balboni TA, et al: Place of death: correlations with quality of life of patients with cancer and predictors of bereaved caregivers' mental health. J Clin Oncol 28(29), 4457–4464, 2010 20837950

Yaghmour NA, Brigham TP, Richter T, et al: Causes of death of residents in ACGME-accredited programs 2000 through 2014: implications for the learning environment. Acad Med 92(7):976–983, 2017 28514230

Ye YG, Davidson JE, Kim K, Zisook S: Physician death by suicide in the United States: 2012–2016. J Psychiatr Res 134:158–165, 2020 33385634

Zisook S, Shear K: Grief and bereavement: what psychiatrists need to know. World
    Psychiatry 8(2):67, 2009
Zisook S, Iglewicz A, Avanzino J, et al: Bereavement: course, consequences, and
    care. Curr Psychiatry Rep 16(10):482, 2014 25135781

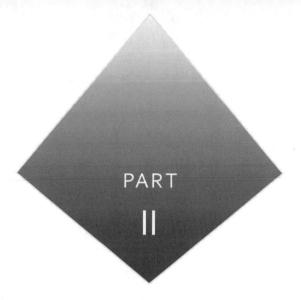

PART

II

Diagnosis and Assessment of Prolonged Grief Disorder

Defining and Diagnosing Prolonged Grief Disorder

Paul K. Maciejewski, Ph.D.
Holly G. Prigerson, Ph.D.

This chapter addresses two fundamental questions about prolonged grief disorder: What is PGD? How does one diagnose it?

The Essence of Prolonged Grief Disorder

We here define *grief* as a constellation of psychologically painful thoughts and feelings evoked by the loss of opportunities for interactions with a *close other* such as a relative, friend, or partner, owing to that person's death. The bereft individual's inability to share and extend mutual interactions, experiences, life narratives, meanings, and common purposes—the loss of "what could have been"—with the close other is inextricably bound with the person's death. Although grief is deeply rooted in a bereft individual's close connection with the decedent developed in the past, grief in bereavement is largely about what is missing in the present and what will be absent in the future.

An individual's experience of loss because of the death of a close other may include a variety of emotions and cognitions. The term *grief* is often applied to the totality of these experiences or equated with sorrow or the intense sadness or pain of loss. But these common notions of grief neglect to capture its distinctive essence. The experience of loss because of the death of a close other is an experience of absence and emptiness, with the concomitant longing or yearning for the richness and sense of coherence, meaning, purpose, place, and wholeness provided by a relationship that is no longer part of one's lived experience.

Prolonged grief is intense grief that is present and persists for an atypically long duration. PGD represents this distressing and disabling experience of prolonged grief. It is worth noting that the pathology of PGD is the result of the persistence and intensity of the grief, and not the presence of unusual or atypical grief symptoms. Intense, even debilitating, grief a short time after a loss is common and to be expected, as the bereft individual has had little time to adapt to a new social circumstance of life in the absence of the close other. Put another way, the typical bereavement response involves intra- and interpersonal readjustment. It often includes a period of emotional turmoil, a sometimes tumultuous process of psychic and social upheaval. This process involves a need to confront how the bereaved survivor will (or will not) attempt to fill the micro-social voids and consequent psychosocial deprivations resulting from the death of the loved one, which we hypothesize will predispose a mourner to PGD (see Figure 4–1) (Maciejewski et al. 2022).

While grief co-travels with most bereft survivors throughout their lives, PGD is different. Intense, debilitating grief that persists beyond a year after a loss has proven to be associated with problematic adjustment to bereavement and a clear indication that the bereft individual has not adapted in a way to promote wellness. We hypothesize that filling the social voids or vacuums created by the significant interpersonal loss will promote a mourner's capacity to lead a life that reinstills a sense of purpose; offers a sense of hope, meaning, and connection; and includes the potential for the future experience of joy, in a world without the decedent. When grief, for whatever reason, remains intense, distressing, and disabling, the mourner becomes stuck in a state of chronic mourning. In this circumstance, the path of grief is a dead end, where PGD is encountered and may endure indefinitely if the psychosocial deprivations created by the loss persist.

Early Conceptualizations of Grief and Grief-Related Psychopathology

Within psychiatry, Sigmund Freud and John Bowlby articulated early and influential ideas about typical ("normal") and pathological forms of grief, which stemmed from their psychoanalytic theories of love and attachment. Other psychiatrists, such as Erich Lindemann and C. Murray Parkes, described clinical characterizations and classifications of somatic, psycholog-

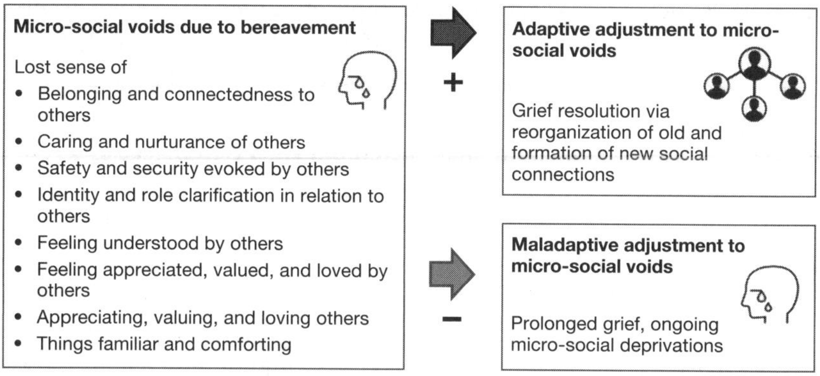

Figure 4–1. Conceptual model relating micro-social voids to bereavement adjustment.

Source. Adapted from a conceptual model advanced in Maciejewski et al. 2022.

ical, and behavioral symptoms and patterns of grief expressed in bereaved individuals. Here we survey the views of these four figures on grief and grief-related psychopathology as they pertain to the origins of PGD.

Freud's "Mourning and Melancholia," 1917

In "Mourning and Melancholia," Freud (1957) articulated the first psychiatric characterization that distinguished "normal" from "pathological" grief. For Freud, grief was considered a normal emotion expressed in mourning; by contrast, melancholia was the pathological form grief took when mourning went awry. Mourning and melancholia, in Freud's view, were both responses to "object loss," with mourning representing a healthy, adaptive process of detachment and melancholia a chronic and destructive response to the loss of the loved object.

Freud described melancholia as a state in which the mourner experienced a "profoundly painful dejection, abrogation of interest in the outside world, loss of the capacity to love, inhibition of all activity, and a lowering of the self-regarding feelings to a degree that finds utterance in self-reproaches" (Freud 1957, p. 125). These symptoms of melancholia resemble many of those currently attributed to or associated with depression. Thus, in his juxtaposition of mourning and melancholia, Freud in essence formulated a view that has prevailed within psychiatry that grief (mourning) in bereavement is normal and depression (melancholia) in bereavement is pathological.

Although the essence of Freud's melancholia has rightfully been interpreted as depression, some elements appear to be more specific to grief. For example, Freud believed that the melancholic mourner was prone to hallucinate about a reunion with the deceased person. Some bereft individuals report experiencing hallucinations in which they hear or see the deceased person talk to or stand before them (Prigerson et al. 1995b). Setting hallucinations aside, it is not uncommon for bereft individuals to engage in reveries about reuniting with the deceased person and, consciously or unconsciously, avoid reminders of the reality of their death. Many bereft individuals struggle with recognizing that their loved one is truly and permanently gone and no longer among the living.

Although Freud described the emotional pain that resulted from the unavailability of the love object both in mourning and in melancholia, he asserted that melancholia featured ambivalence displayed in the melancholic mourner's conflict between withdrawing and maintaining an emotional connection to the deceased person. This conflict might manifest itself as painful yearning for the deceased person, which is the defining feature of grief and PGD. Ambivalence might also find expression in grief-related symptoms of emotional detachment from others, identity confusion in the absence of the deceased person, and avoidance of reminders of the death, all representing the protest against accepting the permanent separation from a loved one.

Lindemann's Normal and Pathognomonic Symptoms for Grief, 1944

Lindemann, a German psychiatrist, also contributed to conceptualizations of pathological grief. Although he did not formally propose diagnostic criteria, he did make important contributions to defining the symptoms, phases, and management of grief based on his clinical experience as a psychiatrist at Massachusetts General Hospital (MGH) in Boston. Lindemann drew his conclusions about normal and pathological grief reactions from his observations of the mentally ill patients he treated who became bereaved relatives of those who died at MGH, relatives of soldiers who died in war, and bereaved survivors of those who died in the Cocoanut Grove fire in Boston (Lindemann 1944).

In describing symptoms of "normal grief," Lindemann wrote:

> The picture shown by persons in acute grief is remarkably uniform. Common to all is the following syndrome: sensations of somatic distress occurring in waves lasting from twenty minutes to an hour at a time, a feeling of tightness in the throat, choking with shortness of breath, need for sighing,

and an empty feeling in the abdomen, lack of muscular power, and an intense subjective distress described as tension or mental pain. (Lindemann 1944, p. 143)

Lindemann's waves of discomfort resembled what Parkes would later referred to as the "pangs of grief": transient, intense feelings of pining for the lost person accompanied by intense anxiety, which Parkes claimed were most common in the second phase of grief after the initial shock and disbelief had subsided (Parkes 1998). Lindemann noted that these pangs of grief could be precipitated by triggers such as the mere mention of the deceased, and resulted in what he described as "a tendency to avoid the syndrome at any cost, to refuse visits lest they should precipitate the reaction, and to keep deliberately from thought all references to the deceased" (Lindemann 1944, p. 141). Lindemann's observation of a "tendency to avoid the syndrome" may be related to the fact that many of his patients were bereaved by traumatic causes such as war and fire. This aspect of Lindemann's characterization of grief also resembles Freud's notion of the melancholic mourner's conflicted feelings about acknowledging the loved one's death.

Lindemann described features of a normal grief response as including 1) conspicuous sighing, especially when asked to discuss the grief; 2) complaints about weakness or extreme fatigue; and 3) digestive problems (e.g., loss of appetite and taste). He described altered sensations, disorientation, and emotional detachment (e.g., "a slight sense of unreality, a feeling of increased emotional distance from other people... [and] intense preoccupation with the image of the deceased") (Lindemann 1944, p. 142). Along with these sensations, Lindemann added a sense of guilt regarding things the mourner could have or should have done to prevent the tragedy as well as a "loss of warmth in relationship to other people [and] a tendency to respond with irritability and anger" (Lindemann 1944, p. 142).

Although Lindemann considered those symptoms to represent normal grief, they appear to overlap considerably with the symptoms he claimed were "pathognomonic for grief" (Lindemann 1944, p. 142). He described pathological grief as having five characteristics: "1) somatic distress, 2) preoccupation with the image of the deceased, 3) guilt, 4) hostile reactions, and 5) loss of patterns of conduct" (i.e., usual ways of behaving) (Lindemann 1944, p. 142). For Lindemann, it was more the intensity of the symptoms and their persistence despite time elapsing from the loss which separated normal grief from pathological grief. In this way, his conceptualization of pathological grief aligns closely with that of PGD: seemingly normal symptoms of grief (e.g., preoccupation with the deceased) may be pathological if they are intense, fail to resolve over time (as they do in typical grief) (Maciejewski et al. 2007), and contribute to significant dysfunction (Prigerson et al. 2009).

Bowlby's Pathological Mourning and Childhood Mourning, 1963

Bowlby, a British developmental psychologist and psychiatrist, is perhaps best known for introducing and developing attachment theory. This theory rested on the notion that infants and very young children have an innate need to establish close emotional bonds with a caregiver (prototypically a mother or mother figure). Bowlby also made seminal contributions to an understanding of mourning, including pathological mourning. Indeed, Bowlby's ideas about grief and mourning in relation to the loss (death) of a person to whom one was closely attached stem from his insights into childhood separation anxiety derived from observations of responses of young children to temporary separation from their caregivers (primarily mothers). According to Bowlby, childhood separation anxiety proceeds through three interrelated phases: *protest*, marked by acute distress and desperate attempts (e.g., crying) to summon the presence of the absent mother figure; *despair*, marked by a hopeless, withdrawn preoccupation with the absent mother figure, inactivity, and what appears to be a state of mourning; and *detachment*, marked by disinterest in the absent mother figure when she returns and greater openness to the surrounding environment and acceptance of care from others (Bowlby 1960). The phase theory of grief of Bowlby and Parkes (1970)—which postulates that grief proceeds from 1) shock and numbness to 2) yearning and searching to 3) disorganization and despair to 4) reorganization and recovery (all described in greater detail later)—has clear roots in form and content in Bowlby's phase theory of childhood separation anxiety.

Like Lindemann, Bowlby considered the inability to arrive at the final stage of normal grief—that is, to relinquish persistent yearning for the attachment figure, accept the loss, and emotionally attach to others—indicative of pathological mourning. More specifically, the four types of pathological mourning Bowlby proposed in 1963 included 1) a persistent yearning to recover the lost object, 2) a persistent anger at both others and the self, 3) compulsive caring for another bereaved person with whom they identified, and 4) denial of the reality of the loss (Bowlby 1963). For Bowlby, the adult mourner's unresolved rage and protest over the loss of the "love object" was the essence of pathological mourning. While the focus on unresolved feelings toward the deceased resembles Freudian conceptualizations of melancholia, Bowlby differed from Freud in that he did not consider pathological grief to be a result of unacknowledged hatred of, or ambivalence toward, the lost love object. Instead, Bowlby considered pathological grief as rooted in self-hatred. In other words, the abandonment by the love object was internalized as a rejection of the self (not the other), a degradation of the ego, and hence diminished self-worth. As in Freud's theory, low self-esteem, despair, and lack of what Bowlby termed "reintegration," the final stage of grief, defined a melancholic, or pathological, response to loss.

Parkes's Typical and Chronic Grief, 1965, and Four Phases of Grief, 1972/1983

Parkes, a British psychiatrist and protégé of Bowlby, devoted his career to a better understanding of bereavement and the care of bereft individuals. Perhaps more than anyone, he laid a solid foundation for and contributed to the emergence of PGD as a diagnostic entity (Prigerson et al. 2009). Unlike Bowlby, whose work had deep theoretical roots in the psychoanalytic tradition and focused primarily on issues related to attachment in early childhood development, Parkes procured and developed insights about grief from clinical observations of bereft adults. Among Parkes's many contributions to the field of bereavement, and most relevant to present-day conceptualizations of PGD, are his characterization and classification of grief and its variants among bereaved psychiatric patients (Parkes 1965a, 1965b) and his (and colleagues') landmark insight and conceptual model of grief as a process that typically proceeds through a series of well-characterized phases (Bowlby and Parkes 1970; Parkes 1972; Parkes and Weiss 1983).

Parkes recognized that there are typical and atypical, or uncomplicated and complicated, forms of grieving (Parkes 1965a). According to Parkes,

> Typical grief is characterized by the onset, after a brief period of numbness, of attacks of yearning and anxiety alternating with longer periods of depression and despair. The sufferer is preoccupied with thoughts of the dead person.... These features... soon begin to decline in intensity, although they may return from time to time at anniversaries or other reminders of the loss. (Parkes 1965b, p. 14)

Parkes also noted that the most common form of atypical grief in his bereaved psychiatric patient sample was chronic grief, which he characterized as follows:

> In [chronic grief] all the usual features of [typical] grief are present...and some or all of them tend to be particularly pronounced. The [chronic grief] reaction is always prolonged and the general impression is one of deep and

pressing sorrow....[Patients with chronic grief] are repeatedly over-whelmed by their yearning and despair. (Parkes 1965b, p. 14)

In essence, Parkes's 1965 characterizations of typical and chronic grief would be fair conceptualizations of what are taken to be typical and pro-longed grief reactions today, with symptoms differing between the two pri-marily in intensity and duration, but not in kind.

Parkes also understood that grief is a process that typically (but not in all cases) proceeds through a series of phases, some of which may repeat, characterized by the following features: 1) shock and numbness, 2) yearning and searching, 3) disorganization and despair, and 4) reorganization and re-covery (Parkes 1972; Parkes and Weiss 1983). In the shock and numbness phase of grief (phase 1), typically experienced immediately after the death of a close other, the bereft individual is emotionally and cognitively stunned by, and exhibits an incapacity to process emotions or information about, the loss. That is, the bereft individual is initially traumatized by the loss of the close other. In the yearning and searching phase of grief (phase 2), the bereft individual longs for the now-inaccessible relationship/deceased person and seeks to retain (hold on to) or recover (find) the relationship/person that was lost. Yearning for the lost person/relationship, the most characteristi-cally defining signature of grief, is the core feature of this second phase of grief. The bereft individual may also experience elements of separation anx-iety, such as an unwillingness to let the deceased close other "go," a period of protest.

In the disorganization and despair phase of grief (phase 3), the bereft in-dividual experiences a growing awareness of and paralysis due to the unset-tling reality of the loss and concomitant hopelessness and elements of depression. Ultimately, in the reorganization and recovery phase of grief (phase 4), the bereft individual is presumed to be at peace with the loss and charts a new path in life without the decedent.

Origins and Evolution of PGD

Although Parkes had developed an exquisite understanding of grief and its "complicated" variants, he did not consider grief in any of its forms to be a mental disorder. Indeed, the broadly accepted conventional wisdom within psychiatry up until the mid-1990s was that pathological aspects of "compli-cated" grief could be attributed to depression, anxiety, posttraumatic stress, or other known forms of psychopathology and not to grief. That is, psychi-atrists generally took complicated grief to be grief (presumed normal) com-plicated by the presence of another syndrome and not as a mental disorder in its own right. Thus, in an important sense, this once-common notion of "complicated grief" is diametrically opposed to PGD as it is understood today.

In the early 1990s, researchers at the University of Pittsburgh launched an effort, spearheaded by Holly Prigerson, to determine whether "complicated" grief might be best understood solely in terms of grief (apart from depression or other known forms of psychopathology) and as a mental disorder in its own right. In a series of original research studies published between 1995 and 1997 in the *American Journal of Psychiatry*, Prigerson and colleagues found that "complicated grief" 6 months after the loss was distinct from bereavement-related depression and anxiety (Prigerson et al. 1995a, 1996) and predictive of mental and physical morbidity 13–25 months after the loss (Prigerson et al. 1995a, 1997). Thus, the studies demonstrated that some form of grief is not benign, providing evidence of a grief disorder. At about the same time, Prigerson and colleagues, including Paul Maciejewski and Charles F. Reynolds, also developed and introduced the Inventory of Complicated Grief (ICG) (Prigerson et al. 1995b), a scale to measure maladaptive symptoms of loss, which became widely used in subsequent studies of complicated grief.

In light of the newly emerging evidence that complicated grief was a distinct, distressing, and disabling psychological syndrome, there were two prominent, early, independent efforts to formulate diagnostic criteria for a new grief-specific disorder. In 1997, Horowitz and colleagues proposed and evaluated diagnostic criteria for "complicated grief disorder," characterized as a stress response syndrome. Around the same time, in 1996, the Pittsburgh group convened a panel of experts in reactions to loss and trauma and the formulation of psychiatric diagnostic criteria to draw up tentative consensus criteria for diagnosing disordered, complicated grief. In 1999, recognizing complicated grief as a trauma-related stress response syndrome, Prigerson and colleagues proposed and evaluated that panel's consensus criteria for complicated grief as criteria for "traumatic grief" (Prigerson et al. 1999). Both Horowitz et al.'s *complicated grief disorder* and Prigerson et al.'s *traumatic grief*, despite differences in name and details for diagnosis, identified and addressed essentially the same diagnostic construct. Thus, by the end of the 1990s, there was agreement among some experts within the scientific community that a distinct variant of grief may well be a mental disorder.

Research in the 2000s continued to build evidence in support of more general recognition of a distinct variant of grief as a mental disorder. Prominently, in a randomized controlled trial published in 2005, Shear and colleagues demonstrated that a psychotherapy treatment tailored to address complicated grief (Complicated Grief Treatment) was significantly more effective than interpersonal psychotherapy in the reduction and rate of reduction of symptoms of complicated grief among bereaved individuals who met criteria for complicated grief (Shear et al. 2005). The study clearly established that this grief disorder was amenable to treatment, so its entry into ICD and DSM would likely facilitate and broaden the use and development of effective treatments.

In a study published in 2009, Prigerson and colleagues (including Horowitz, Parkes, Maciejewski, Maercker, Jacobs, Bonanno, Boelen, and other internationally renowned experts on grief in bereavement) developed, evaluated, and proposed for inclusion in DSM-5-TR and ICD-11 robust diagnostic criteria for a disorder of grief that they named *prolonged grief disorder* (Prigerson et al. 2009). This study, sponsored by the National Institute of Mental Health and designed specifically to evaluate diagnostic criteria for disordered grief, included a systematic and comprehensive assessment of both symptom items and diagnostic algorithms in the construction of specific, sensitive, and efficient diagnostic criteria for PGD. Prigerson et al.'s proposal for PGD became the impetus and foundation for PGD's admission to ICD-11 and DSM-5-TR (American Psychiatric Association 2022; World Health Organization 2022).

Diagnostic Criteria for PGD

ICD-11 Diagnostic Guideline for PGD

A German-Swiss psychiatrist with expertise in traumatic stress response syndromes, Andreas Maercker, was chair of the ICD-11 Workgroup on Stress-Associated Disorders. He had worked with Horowitz, Prigerson, and Maciejewski on studies of PGD and was familiar with the evidence in support of it as a distinct new form of psychiatric illness (Maciejewski et al. 2016; Prigerson et al. 2009). Maercker considered the available evidence for PGD sufficiently compelling to recommend its inclusion as an official additional mental disorder in ICD-11 (Maercker et al. 2013; World Health Organization 2022). In 2013, he wrote:

> Prolonged grief disorder is a new diagnosis being proposed for ICD-11, which describes abnormally persistent and disabling responses to bereavement. It is defined as a severe and enduring symptom pattern of yearning or longing for the deceased or a persistent preoccupation with the deceased. This reaction may be associated with difficulties accepting the death, feelings of loss of a part of oneself, anger about the loss, [and] guilt. (Maercker et al. 2013, p. 202)

He went on to note that studies from Western and Eastern cultures had supported the validity of these criteria, and he asserted that it was time to recognize PGD as a distinctive mental disorder. The decision was made to include the disorder in ICD-11, using the name *prolonged grief disorder* and referencing *PLoS Medicine* (Prigerson et al. 2009) for empirical evidence in support of the proposed criteria.

The ICD-11 guideline for the diagnosis of PGD relies primarily on the clinical judgment of (mental) health care professionals to grasp the concept of PGD and identify a few of its essential features in bereaved individuals to make a diagnosis. ICD-11's description and required features for making a diagnosis of PGD are presented in Table 4–1. Whereas the ICD-11 formulation of criteria for PGD retained the primacy of yearning for and preoccupation with the deceased and used the 6-month postloss timing criterion validated in *PLoS Medicine* (Prigerson et al. 2009), it departed in a few important ways. For example, the ICD-11 PGD criteria require only any one of 10 additional symptoms, some of which had not yet been empirically tested. Killikelly and Maercker (2017) have argued that this simpler, "gestalt" approach to diagnostic classification is more flexible and clinically useful, and that it facilitates cross-cultural application (Stelzer et al. 2020) in ways that the more structured DSM approach does not.

Eisma et al. (2020) critiqued the ICD-11 PGD criteria for the challenges they pose to researchers. They faulted the ICD-11 PGD criteria for including symptoms such as "guilt," "blame," and "the inability to experience positive emotions" that had not been validated in prior criteria sets. They criticized the use of single-word symptoms such as "guilt," "anger," "denial," and "blame," as they lack specificity and could be subject to multiple interpretations: "For example, 'blame' could refer to self-blame or other-blame, blame for the death, or blame for something else. Since self-blame is much more prevalent in bereaved persons than blaming others the interpretation of this criterion influences its prevalence" (Eisma et al. 2020, p. 2, citation removed). Another problematic symptom in the ICD-11 PGD criteria concerns the item "denial." It is unclear how to assess and evaluate denial given that acknowledgment of denial suggests an awareness that belies it. Thus ICD's impressionistic nature of diagnosing PGD enables clinicians to apply the criteria as they see fit, leaving more to their discretion than would checking symptoms off criterion lists, but there have been issues taken with the symptoms identified in ICD-11's characterization and with the lack of specificity of the symptom assessments.

Beyond issues with the symptoms included in the ICD-11 PGD criteria, concerns have been raised regarding the minimal requirements for meeting

Table 4–1.   ICD-11 prolonged grief disorder (ICD-11 code: 6B42)

Description

Prolonged grief disorder is a disturbance in which, following the death of a partner, parent, child, or other person close to the bereaved, there is a persistent and pervasive grief response characterized by longing for the deceased or persistent preoccupation with the deceased accompanied by intense emotional pain (e.g. sadness, guilt, anger, denial, blame, difficulty accepting the death, feeling one has lost a part of one's self, an inability to experience positive mood, emotional numbness, difficulty in engaging with social or other activities). The grief response has persisted for an atypically long period of time following the loss (more than 6 months at a minimum) and clearly exceeds expected social, cultural, or religious norms for the individual's culture and context. Grief reactions that have persisted for longer periods that are within a normative period of grieving given the person's cultural and religious context are viewed as normal bereavement responses and are not assigned a diagnosis. The disturbance causes significant impairment in personal, family, social, educational, occupational, or other important areas of functioning.

Diagnostic requirements: essential (required) features

- History of bereavement following the death of a partner, parent, child, or other person close to the bereaved.
- A persistent and pervasive grief response characterized by longing for the deceased or persistent preoccupation with the deceased accompanied by intense emotional pain. This may be manifested by experiences such as sadness, guilt, anger, denial, blame, difficulty accepting the death, feeling one has lost a part of one's self, an inability to experience positive mood, emotional numbness, and difficulty in engaging with social or other activities.
- The pervasive grief response has persisted for an atypically long period of time following the loss, markedly exceeding expected social, cultural, or religious norms for the individual's culture and context. Grief responses lasting for less than 6 months, and for longer periods in some cultural contexts, should not be regarded as meeting this requirement.
- The disturbance results in significant impairment in personal, family, social, educational, occupational, or other important areas of functioning. If functioning is maintained, it is only through significant additional effort.

Source.   https://icd.who.int/browse11/l-m/en#/http://id.who.int/icd/entity/ 1183832314

diagnostic criteria and multiple ways in which they could be met (e.g., en-dorsing any of 10 symptoms) (Eisma et al. 2020). Not only have these been shown to increase the prevalence rates for PGD, but Eisma et al. (2020) claimed that they could also result in overdiagnosis (i.e., false-positive diag-noses). The laxity of the diagnostic criteria and multiple ways to meet them for an ICD-11 PGD diagnosis hinder generalizability and comparison across individuals, samples, and studies. In these ways, the ICD-11 formulation poses challenges to establishing uniform and agreed-on criteria (i.e., standardization) for a PGD diagnosis. Too much discretion of the clinician may open the door to the possibility of comparing apples with oranges.

DSM-5-TR Diagnostic Criteria for PGD

As ICD-11 moved forward with inclusion of PGD as an official diagnosis, efforts to harmonize criteria between diagnostic manuals put pressure on DSM to do the same. In its 2013 release (DSM-5) (American Psychiatric Association 2013), the editors placed what they called *persistent complex bereavement disorder* (PCBD) in Section III (its Appendix) as an "emerging diagnosis" (Friedman 2016). Matthew Friedman, chair of the DSM-5 Workgroup on Trauma- and Stress-Related and Dissociative Disorders, wrote in the *American Journal of Psychiatry*,

> Although the DSM-5 sub-workgroup was very favorably disposed toward adding a new diagnosis addressing abnormal bereavement-related emotions and behavior…it seemed apparent that more research was needed before data supporting specific diagnostic criteria for a bereavement-related disorder could satisfy DSM-5's rigorous standards for inclusion of a new diagnosis. (Friedman 2016, p. 864)

Once the ICD-11 editors had considered the evidence sufficient to justify including PGD, the DSM editors considered it time to reevaluate their position. Regardless of the pros and cons of the ICD-11 criteria for PGD, there is no doubt that by including PGD as a new mental disorder, ICD-11 led DSM in advancing formal medical recognition of this diagnosis.

Next we describe the DSM-5-TR editors' reaction to ICD's decision. In June 2019, the DSM-5-TR Workgroup led by Paul Appelbaum[1] held a meeting in New York City that invited relevant thought-leaders in psychiatric diagnosis to discuss the evidence in support of a bereavement-related disorder. Present were the two leading research groups on bereavement in adults (Shear and Reynolds; Prigerson and Maciejewski) and experts in child bereavement (Robert Pynoos and Christopher Layne). Prigerson and Maciejewski presented data in support of PGD's inclusion, Reynolds presented

---

[1] The workgroup included Philip Wang, David Brent, Kenneth Kendler, Thomas Widiger, Ellen Leibenluft, Katharine Phillips, Roberto Lewis, Kimberly Yonkers, Michael First, and Saul Levin.

case histories of bereaved adults whom his team had diagnosed with PGD, and Layne and Pynoos presented their data on child responses to bereavement. At the end of the meeting, committee members drafted provisional criteria based on these presentations. The research groups were then tasked with evaluating the provisional criteria using extant data. Prigerson and Maciejewski, Shear and Reynolds, and Pynoos and Layne submitted their analyses to the committee in September 2019. The Steering Committee reviewed the data and approved inclusion of a provisional PGD criteria set in Section II of DSM.

There was then a public commentary period from April 6 to May 20, 2020, in which reactions to the proposed PGD criteria set were invited at the American Psychiatric Association (APA) website. More than 53 pages of public comments were submitted to the APA online portal. One of the main concerns expressed in the public comments related to pathologizing normal grief reactions. Several commentators expressed appreciation for delaying the diagnosis of PGD until at least 12 months had elapsed since the death; this was a change from PCBD's requirement of only 6 months. This 6-month deferment appeared to reduce concerns about prematurely pathologizing grief.

The DSM criteria set for PGD also differed from PCBD in that it required three of eight "C Criteria" be met for a diagnosis; it also focused more on "yearning for" the deceased and less on "preoccupation with the circumstances of the death" among adults (the latter of which could be captured by a PTSD diagnosis), although that was retained for children. (Note that we focus in this chapter on PGD criteria for adults only. Chapters 2 and 3 address bereavement and PGD criteria for children.)

The DSM-5-TR diagnostic criteria for PGD are presented in Box 4–1. To receive a diagnosis of PGD, an individual must meet the following requirements: Criterion A, be bereaved owing to the death of a close other that occurred at least 12 months ago (for children and adolescents, at least 6 months ago); Criterion B, experience defining, core symptoms of grief, i.e., yearning for and/or preoccupation with thoughts of the deceased person nearly every day, for at least the last month; Criterion C, experience at least three of eight other symptoms of grief to a clinically significant degree nearly every day for at least the last month; and Criterion D, experience this grief as the cause of clinically significant distress or impairment in social, occupational, or other important areas of functioning. In addition, the duration and severity of the bereavement reaction must clearly exceed expected social, cultural, or religious norms for the individual's culture and context (Criterion E) and must not be better attributed to another mental, behavioral, or physical health condition (Criterion F).

Box 4–1. Prolonged Grief Disorder

F43.81

A. The death, at least 12 months ago, of a person who was close to the bereaved individual (for children and adolescents, at least 6 months ago).
B. Since the death, the development of a persistent grief response characterized by one or both of the following symptoms, which have been present most days to a clinically significant degree. In addition, the symptom(s) has occurred nearly every day for at least the last month:

 1. Intense yearning/longing for the deceased person.
 2. Preoccupation with thoughts or memories of the deceased person (in children and adolescents, preoccupation may focus on the circumstances of the death).

C. Since the death, at least three of the following symptoms have been present most days to a clinically significant degree. In addition, the symptoms have occurred nearly every day for at least the last month:

 1. Identity disruption (e.g., feeling as though part of oneself has died) since the death.
 2. Marked sense of disbelief about the death.
 3. Avoidance of reminders that the person is dead (in children and adolescents, may be characterized by efforts to avoid reminders).
 4. Intense emotional pain (e.g., anger, bitterness, sorrow) related to the death.
 5. Difficulty reintegrating into one's relationships and activities after the death (e.g., problems engaging with friends, pursuing interests, or planning for the future).
 6. Emotional numbness (absence or marked reduction of emotional experience) as a result of the death.
 7. Feeling that life is meaningless as a result of the death.
 8. Intense loneliness as a result of the death.

D. The disturbance causes clinically significant distress or impairment in social, occupational, or other important areas of functioning.
E. The duration and severity of the bereavement reaction clearly exceed expected social, cultural, or religious norms for the individual's culture and context.
F. The symptoms are not better explained by another mental disorder, such as major depressive disorder or posttraumatic stress disorder, and are not attributable to the physiological effects of a substance (e.g., medication, alcohol) or another medical condition.

Source. Reprinted from American Psychiatric Association: Diagnostic and Statistical Manual of Mental Disorders, 5th Edition, Text Revision, Washington, DC, American Psychiatric Association, 2022. Copyright © 2022 American Psychiatric Association. Used with permission.

Diagnostic Classification of PGD

ICD-11 and DSM-5-TR classify PGD as a stress response syndrome under the headings "Disorders Specifically Associated With Stress" and "Trauma- and Stressor-Related Disorders," respectively. This similar classification of PGD in ICD-11 and DSM-5-TR reflects a common goal for better alignment and harmonization between the ICD-11 and DSM-5 classifications of mental disorders (Regier et al. 2013).

Although PGD has been placed within the existing classification systems for ICD-11 and DSM-5-TR, there is a need for further research, exploration, and understanding of PGD to confirm PGD's most appropriate diagnostic home. For example, is PGD best considered a stress response syndrome? An adjustment or attachment disorder? Or, as data from a review of PGD's neurobiological correlates would suggest (Kakarala et al. 2020), a consequence of reward system dysfunction akin to an addictive disorder? The diagnostic home of PGD may also suggest which interventions may most effectively treat it. For example, to the extent that PGD is shown to be the result of reward system dysfunction, novel treatments such as naltrexone may prove effective although antidepressant treatments have not (Reynolds et al. 1999). Consistent with a microsociological theory of adaptation to loss (Maciejewski et al. 2022), interventions that free mourners from the grip of grief—e.g., either biochemically by making a focus on the deceased person less "rewarding" (Gang et al. 2021) or cognitively by restructuring negative thoughts that may impede interest and efforts to interact with others—may open patients to the possibility of gratifying interpersonal connections, which might effectively reduce symptoms of PGD. We acknowledge that, although these conceptual models and novel treatments offer promise, they await formal testing and confirmation. We refer readers to Chapter 7 for a thorough discussion of proven treatments for PGD.

Instruments for Assessing PGD

The Prolonged Grief-13-Revised Scale

The Prolonged Grief-13-Revised scale (PG-13-R, which can be found in Appendix A) (Prigerson et al. 2021a) is a 13-item instrument that can be used for the dual purposes of assessing grief intensity continuously on a dimensional scale and of diagnosing PGD according to the DSM-5-TR criteria. Its predecessor, the PG-13 (Prigerson and Maciejewski 2008), served the same purposes and can be used to diagnose PGD according to the criteria originally proposed for PGD's inclusion in DSM-5 and ICD-11 (Prigerson et al. 2009). Items in the PG-13 are a subset of those in the Inventory of Complicated Grief – Revised (ICG-R) (Prigerson and Jacobs 2001), a revision of ICG (Prigerson et al. 1995b). Items included in the PG-13 were those found to be informative and unbiased with respect to sex, relationship to the decedent, and time since the loss in item response theory–based item analysis and that mapped onto our criteria for PGD proposed in 2009 (Prigerson et al. 2009). In essence, PG-13-R is an updated version of PG-13 in which the items in the scale match the items required to assess PGD using the DSM-5-TR criteria (Box 4–1). The PG-13-R items assess bereavement by and time since the death of the close other (Items 1 and 2; DSM-5-TR Criterion A), core defining symptoms of grief (Items 3 and 4; DSM-5-TR Criterion B), other grief symptoms (Items 5–12; DSM-5-TR Criterion C), and grief-related impairment (Item 13; DSM-5-TR Criterion D).

We developed and used the PG-13-R to evaluate the DSM-5-TR criteria for PGD using data from investigations conducted at Yale University ($N=270$), Utrecht University ($N=163$), and Oxford University ($N=239$) (Prigerson et al. 2021a). Results indicated that the grief symptoms assessed using the PG-13-R were internally consistent (Cronbach's $\alpha=0.83$, 0.90, and 0.93, for Yale, Utrecht, and Oxford, respectively). The DSM-5-TR PGD diagnosis was shown to be distinguishable from PTSD ($\phi=0.12$), major depressive disorder (MDD; $\phi=0.25$), and generalized anxiety disorder (GAD) ($\phi=0.26$) at the baseline assessments, which occurred 12–24 months after the death. Temporal stability between the baseline assessments and follow-up (average of 5.3–12 months later) was remarkable for this diagnosis ($r=0.86$, $P<0.001$) and superior to the temporal stability demonstrated for the other disorders (e.g., $r=0.31$, $P=0.030$ for MDD; $r=-0.07$, $P=0.653$ for GAD; PTSD was inestimable because only one study participant met criteria for PTSD at the follow-up assessment). The differences in temporal stability between the PGD and MDD diagnoses suggests that PGD symptomatology is more chronic and MDD and the other disorders are more episodic.

Both the DSM PGD diagnosis and the PG-13-R symptom summary score at baseline were statistically significantly associated ($P<0.05$) with symptoms and diagnoses of PTSD, MDD, and GAD, suicidal ideation, worse quality of life, and functional impairments at baseline and follow-up in the Yale, Utrecht, and Oxford datasets. Overall, the newly proposed DSM criteria for PGD and the PG-13-R both proved to be reliable and valid measures for the classification of bereaved individuals with maladaptive grief responses. The prevalence rates in these community-based bereaved samples at ~1 year after the loss using the DSM-5-TR PGD criteria were 4%–15%—rates low enough to reduce concerns that the DSM-proposed criteria would diagnose typical grief as pathological. Prevalence rates would be expected to be higher among treatment-seeking individuals.

Research is needed to determine the extent to which self-report and interview-based assessments of grief and PGD using the PG-13-R measure agree with clinical diagnoses of PGD. Research is also needed to validate the DSM-5-TR PGD criteria in different countries, cultures, circumstances of death (e.g., suicide, homicide, natural disaster, human causation, natural causes), racial and ethnic groups, gender identities, and ages of the deceased and the survivors.

The Structured Clinical Interview for PGD (SCIP)

SCIP (which can be found in Appendix B) is a structured clinical interview designed to be administered by mental health professionals to facilitate clinical assessment and diagnosis of PGD. Guided by the SCIP script, interviewers gather information from bereaved individuals that is relevant to and sufficient for a diagnostic assessment for PGD based on a sequence of questions/prompts and related clinical judgments. In particular, SCIP facilitates clinical consideration of grief-related impairments in functioning (such as social and occupational; DSM-5-TR Criterion D), cultural norms and expectations related to grief and mourning (DSM-5-TR Criterion E), and differential diagnosis (DSM-5-TR Criterion F) in the clinical assessment for PGD. It is currently being used as a primary outcome in a randomized controlled trial of naltrexone (Gang et al. 2021) and multiple other studies.

Clinical Utility of a Prolonged Grief Disorder Diagnosis

It is crucially important to determine whether PGD, as a newly defined mental disorder, is clinically useful. According to First (2010), a mental disorder definition with clinical utility facilitates communication, promotes effective interventions, predicts management needs and outcomes, and differentiates disorders from nondisorders, as well as from comorbid disorders.

Criteria

As mentioned earlier, Killikelly and Maercker (2017) claimed that ICD-11 criteria for PGD had the advantage over PCBD (DSM-5) with respect to clinical utility. In their words:

> The new PGD ICD-11 criteria are conceptualized in line with the key aims of the WHO to improve clinical utility and international applicability. Historically, the revision of diagnostic manuals such as the DSM and ICD has centered on improving the diagnostic specification and reliability of disorder criteria.... [T]he long and, at times, complicated symptom lists and categories are not always practical in the clinical setting.... To establish the clinical utility...the ICD revision group adopted a two-phase research strategy: 1) to develop guidelines for the formative structure and content of a mental disorder; and 2) to evaluate the usability of these guidelines in reaching diagnostic decisions in the international field. (Killikelly and Maercker 2017, p. 4)

In essence, Maercker and Killikelly asserted that the ICD-11 formulation was easier to apply because it was shorter and less structured, which they suggested made it easier to adapt to a variety of settings. Cozza et al. (2020) have also focused on the need to optimize the clinical utility of criteria for PGD, noting that ICD-11 performed well in this regard and that the ICD criteria were less restrictive than the DSM-5 criteria for PCBD.

A separate study (Lichtenthal et al. 2018) supported by the National Institute of Mental Health was designed to examine the clinical utility of the PGD criteria as outlined in *PLoS Medicine* (Prigerson et al. 2009). The study involved an initial survey of mental health professionals' attitudes and beliefs about those diagnostic criteria. When asked whether they considered that the criteria 1) were informative for devising a treatment plan; 2) improved communication between clinicians about the client's grief; 3) were easy to use; and 4) enhanced the overall clinical utility of the PGD diagnosis, more than 95% of those surveyed responded "moderately" to "extremely" (Lichtenthal et al. 2018). The study also demonstrated that a very brief tutorial on diagnosis of PGD yielded high rates of diagnostic accuracy while not inflating rates of misdiagnosis, thus helping minimize concerns about pathologizing normal grief reactions.

Differential Diagnosis

The final aspect of clinical utility concerns differential diagnosis: how PGD is distinguished from other established mental disorders that may follow from the death of a close other. Now that the DSM-5-R criteria for PGD have been validated and approved as an official psychiatric diagnosis, clinicians need to know how PGD criteria differ from those of other common mental disorders secondary to bereavement, such as MDD or PTSD. As part of the study to examine the clinical utility of the PGD diagnosis, we formulated typologies to assist clinicians in making a diagnostic determination. We developed virtual standardized patients (VSPs) who were evaluated to determine whether a mental health professional could discern a diagnosis of MDD or PTSD relative to PGD and a case depicting normative grief. (Video clips of these VSPs can be found at https://endoflife.weill.cornell.edu/grief-resources/resources-clinicians.) Here we summarize the distinctions between PGD, MDD, and PTSD among bereaved individuals.

Distinctions between PGD and MDD are summarized in Table 4–2. Whereas PGD focuses on separation distress, MDD is experienced as a pervasively low mood, feeling blue and sad, regardless of the circumstances (e.g., not specific to the loss of a close other). In PGD, yearning, pining, and longing for the deceased person (the "loss object") is a core symptom. Depressive symptoms, per se, do not involve yearning. PGD involves feelings of comfort, security, and safety in response to memories of the deceased person. By contrast, MDD reactions involve an inability to find comfort or joy in the wake of the loss, and the mourner exhibits more of a flat affect. As noted previously, MDD is also more episodic, whereas symptoms of PGD tend to remain intense and unremitting. PGD is specific to the person lost and not generic to other experiences or outcomes that are unrelated to loss. MDD is not exclusively triggered by an interpersonal loss. MDD is *psychological*, an intrapersonal emotional experience that could be triggered by a wide variety of experiences; PGD is *social*, an experience of interpersonal, or social, deprivation (Maciejewski et al. 2022). Mourners with PGD may experience identity disturbance and role confusion, involving questioning whom one is without the deceased person and where one fits into a world without the deceased in it. MDD is associated with diminished feelings of self-esteem and social status, but not a sense of role confusion or diminished sense of self, per se. MDD is associated with a pessimistic view and expectation that bad things will happen. PGD is characterized by a state of disbelief and lack of acceptance of the death.

Distinctions between PGD and PTSD are summarized in Table 4–3. PTSD does not involve an intense yearning for the deceased person or preoccupation with thoughts of the deceased person. Instead, PTSD is a fear-based response to disturbing, intrusive thoughts about a traumatic event. In PGD, thoughts of the deceased person are typically bittersweet, evoking nostalgia and fondness, comfort, security, positive memories, and missing the relationship shared with the deceased person. With PTSD, there is a hypervigilance that involves scanning the environment for potential threats to safety. In PGD, the threat to safety is a result of the absence of the deceased person, who enhanced feelings of safety and self-worth. Rather than pangs of grief indicative of PGD, intrusive thoughts haunt the survivor with PTSD. PTSD results from a traumatic event that may or may not have involved the

Table 4–2.   Differences between PGD and MDD secondary to bereavement

PGD	MDD
Yearning, longing, pining for deceased	Yearning is not characteristic of MDD
Sadness in response to thinking about the loss	Pervasive low mood, sadness
Bittersweet emotions evoked by memories of the deceased	Inability to feel joy or happiness in response to memories of the deceased
Pangs of grief (waves of emotion related to missing the deceased)	Pangs of grief are not characteristic of MDD
Personal—person-specific, response to close other	Not person-specific, pervasive low mood not triggered exclusively by an interpersonal loss
Social—an experience of social, interpersonal deprivation precipitating the need to reconfigure social network	Psychological—an internal, emotional experience
Chronic, persistent state	Episodic; comes and goes
Evokes identity disturbance (questioning sense of self, who one is and where one fits in, roles, feeling unwhole)	Evokes feelings of low self-esteem and self-worth, but not necessarily identity disturbance or role confusion
Disbelief, lack of acceptance of the death	Bad outcomes are expected; expectations are confirmed rather than shattered

death of a significant other; PGD results from the loss of a significant person in the life of the mourner. PGD is, by definition, social, as it is the result of an interpersonal loss, and it engenders social deprivations. PTSD is psychological—an intrapersonal emotional reaction to a threatening event. At the risk of oversimplification: for PTSD, it is a response to the "how" not the "who" of the death, and living in fear that bad things can happen to anyone at any time; for PGD, it is a response to the "who" not the "how" of the death, which evokes a cascade of emotions related to missing the close other.

Common Misconceptions about PGD

Although we have described, and hopefully clarified, the conceptualization of and diagnostic criteria for PGD, we are aware that many misconceptions

Table 4–3.   Differences between PGD and PTSD secondary to bereavement

PGD	PTSD
Yearning, longing, pining for deceased	Yearning is not characteristic of PTSD
Preoccupation with thoughts of deceased, evoking sense of missing	Intrusive thoughts about the death, typically focused on the circumstances of the death
Avoidance of reminders that the deceased is truly gone and permanently unavailable	Avoidance of reminders of the death itself
Bittersweet emotions evoked by memories of the deceased	Memories of death evoke fear and horror
Pangs of grief (waves of emotion related to missing the deceased)	No pangs of grief; unbidden images of the death haunt rather than console
Personal—person-specific, response to close other (the "who" not the "how" of the loss)	Not person-specific but rather event-specific, linked to a psychologically traumatic experience that evokes extreme fear, helplessness, or horror (the "how" not the "who")
Social—an experience of social, interpersonal deprivation	Psychological—an intrapersonal emotional reaction to a traumatic exposure
Hyperfocus, preoccupation with thoughts of deceased; deliberate reminiscing that evokes feelings of safety and security	Hypervigilance regarding potential dangers; unwanted thoughts and fears
Searching for the deceased or imagining seeing the deceased	No searching but keen focus on possible threats to safety
Disengagement and loss of interest in other people	Hyperalert to scan environment for danger; other people perceived as potential threat
Social support system affected	Social support system not necessarily affected

may remain about this diagnosis. Next we address common misunderstandings about PGD.

Misconception 1: PGD Pathologizes Normal Grief

The diagnostic criteria have been applied to several community-based bereaved groups, and the prevalence rate is ~4% in these samples (Prigerson et al. 2009). This means that only about four of a hundred bereaved individuals would meet criteria for PGD. Clearly, the average or statistical norm, or modal response, does not fall into this group, as ~96% do not meet diagnostic criteria for PGD. The overwhelming majority of bereaved individuals would not even meet the symptom threshold for PGD beyond 6 months, let alone 12 months, after the death. As we found in another report in a sample of mostly older adults bereaved by deaths attributed to natural causes that excluded those who met criteria for PGD (Maciejewski et al. 2007), all the negative symptoms of grief were on the decline by 6 months after the death. Thus, it appears that rather than pathologizing normal grief, we are identifying a small subset of mourners who are stuck in a chronically intense, disturbingly disruptive grieving state (Prigerson et al. 2021a).

Misconception 2: PGD Creates False Positives

The diagnostic criteria for PGD included in DSM-5-TR are highly specific. That is, they identify true-positive cases of PGD without many, if any, false positives (e.g., 4 of 268, or 1.5%, in an analysis of PGD criteria in *PLoS Medicine* [Maciejewski et al. 2016]). By contrast, without the diagnosis, bereaved individuals would actually be undetected false negatives (i.e., missed cases) who would be considered well and not significantly distressed or impaired, despite severe distress, dysfunction, and risk of morbid complications of their grief (Prigerson et al. 2021a).

Misconception 3: PGD Stigmatizes Bereaved Individuals

We conducted a study to explore how a bereaved individual would feel if receiving a diagnosis such as PGD. We found that more than 90% of respondents who met criteria for a diagnosis of PGD reported that they would be relieved to know that having such a diagnosis was indicative of a recognizable psychiatric condition, and 100% reported that they would be interested in receiving treatment for their severe grief symptoms (Johnson et al. 2009). These results suggest that bereaved individuals who meet criteria for PGD

welcome the news that there is a disorder that accurately captures their experience and struggles. Further, they reported feeling hopeful that greater
precision in diagnosis would translate to more effective treatment.

Misconception 4: PGD Lacks Clinical Utility

We conducted a study to determine whether mental health professionals
considered the PGD diagnosis clinically useful and whether they could be
readily trained in accurately diagnosing and distinguishing PGD from other
mental disorders common in bereavement (e.g., PTSD and MDD) (Lichtenthal et al. 2018). We found that clinicians who were provided with information about PGD were 4.5 times more likely to diagnose PGD accurately
than those not receiving such information. There were no significant group
differences in the likelihood of clinicians accurately diagnosing normative
grief, MDD, or PTSD, suggesting that the diagnosis did not inflate rates of
pathologizing normal grief. There were significant between-group differences in treatment recommendations for PGD cases. Clinical utility ratings
of the PGD diagnostic criteria were high, with large majorities of clinicians
rating those criteria as easy to use (97%) and overall clinically useful (95%).

Misconception 5: Time Heals Grief So There Is No Need for Intervention

There is a popular adage, "grief never ends, it changes." "Normal" grief does
not conclude at any circumscribed time and, for most of us, is lifelong. But for
those with PGD, it does not change. Although most people adjust to bereavement, not all do (Maciejewski et al. 2007, 2022). We have found that bereaved
individuals who meet PGD criteria often remain stuck in chronically intense-
level symptomatic distress. For example, we found temporal stability of a PGD
diagnosis to be very high across assessments 5–7 months apart ($r=0.86$) compared with other mental disorders secondary to bereavement such as MDD
($r=0.31$) or GAD ($r=-0.07$). Further, we found that grief symptoms were
not responsive to tricyclic antidepressants or interpersonal psychotherapy
(Prigerson et al. 2021b). These results suggest that neither time nor antidepressant treatment is likely to heal the grief of a person diagnosed with PGD.

Misconception 6: Psychiatry Is "Pushing Pills" to Make You Forget Your Deceased Loved One

Medications prescribed for PGD are neither intended nor expected to di-
minish the love of a mourner for the deceased loved one. They are intended
to reduce the sadness, anxiety, and sorrow that can at times prove not only

extremely upsetting but even incapacitating, leaving a mourner to question the desire to live without the deceased person. In the case of naltrexone, some have suggested that it will reduce social connectedness of mourners; in fact, there is no evidence of this—it is more likely, moreover, that the opposite may occur. Researchers are testing the hypothesis that naltrexone can release a mourner from the exclusive focus on the "rewarding" relationship with the deceased person, thereby freeing them to explore relationships with living others. In a very small sample to date, naltrexone has been shown to enhance social interactions rather than reduce them (Gang et al. 2021). The evidence is not yet conclusive, but if naltrexone promotes social connectedness and meaningful relationships with others and reduces symptoms of PGD and suicidal thoughts and behaviors, we think that it should be made known and available to mourners who are struggling, who have not been helped by antidepressants or psychotherapy, and who wish to try it to reduce their struggles with grief.

Conclusion

In this chapter, we define what PGD is, offer our conceptualization of it, and describe its history in the psychiatric literature. We provide a detailed explanation of the various formulations PGD has taken leading up to publication in ICD-11 and DSM-5-TR, and we share PG-13-R, a validated self-report instrument to assess PGD, and SCIP, a structured clinical interview of PGD. We discuss issues related to differential diagnosis and PGD's diagnostic home (i.e., its place among other disorders in DSM) and the implications of the diagnosis and diagnostic categorization for its treatment. We end with a commentary addressing some common misconceptions about PGD.

There may follow understandable and expected concerns about misdiagnosis and mistreatment—as should be when any new diagnostic or clinical entity is introduced, administered, and studied. Despite concerns that have been raised, there is no doubt that having uniform and agreed-on (standardized) diagnostic criteria for PGD is an important first step in advancing understanding of this new diagnostic classification.

References

American Psychiatric Association: Diagnostic and Statistical Manual of Mental Disorders, 5th Edition. Arlington, VA, American Psychiatric Association, 2013

American Psychiatric Association: Diagnostic and Statistical Manual of Mental Disorders, 5th Edition, Text Revision. Washington, DC, American Psychiatric Association, 2022

Bowlby J: Separation anxiety. Int J Psychoanal 41:89–113, 1960 13803480

Bowlby J: Pathological mourning and childhood mourning. J Am Psychoanal Assoc 11:500–541, 1963 14014626

Bowlby J, Parkes CM: Separation and loss within the family, in The Child in His Family: International Yearbook of Child Psychiatry and Allied Professions. Edited by EJ Anthony, C Koupernik. New York, Wiley, 1970, pp 197–216

Cozza SJ, Shear MK, Reynolds CF, et al: Optimizing the clinical utility of four proposed criteria for a persistent and impairing grief disorder by emphasizing core, rather than associated symptoms. Psychol Med 50(3):438–445, 2020 30829195

Eisma MC, Rosner R, Comtesse H: ICD-11 prolonged grief disorder criteria: turning challenges into opportunities with multiverse analyses. Front Psychiatry 11:752, 2020 32848929

First MB: Clinical utility in the revision of the Diagnostic and Statistical Manual of Mental Disorders (DSM). Prof Psychol Res Pr 41(6):465–473, 2010

Freud S: Mourning and melancholia, in A General Selection From the Works of Sigmund Freud. Edited by Rickman J. Garden City, New York, Doubleday Anchor, 1957, pp 124–140

Friedman MJ: Seeking the best bereavement-related diagnostic criteria. Am J Psychiatry 173(9):864–865, 2016 27581694

Gang J, Kocsis J, Avery J, et al: Naltrexone treatment for prolonged grief disorder: study protocol for a randomized, triple-blinded, placebo-controlled trial. Trials 22(1):110, 2021 33522931

Johnson JG, First MB, Block S, et al: Stigmatization and receptivity to mental health services among recently bereaved adults. Death Stud 33(8):691–711, 2009 19697482

Kakarala SE, Roberts KE, Rogers M, et al: The neurobiological reward system in prolonged grief disorder (PGD): a systematic review. Psychiatry Res Neuroimaging 303:111135, 2020 32629197

Killikelly C, Maercker A: Prolonged grief disorder for ICD-11: the primacy of clinical utility and international applicability. Eur J Psychotraumatol 8(Suppl 6):1476441, 2017 29887976

Lichtenthal WG, Maciejewski PK, Demirjian C, et al: Evidence of the clinical utility of a prolonged grief disorder diagnosis. World Psychiatry 17(3):364–365, 2018 30229568

Lindemann E: Symptomatology and management of acute grief. Am J Psychiatry 101:141–148, 1944

Maciejewski PK, Zhang B, Block SD, Prigerson HG: An empirical examination of the stage theory of grief. JAMA 297(7):716–723, 2007 17312291; erratum in JAMA 297(20):2200, 2007

Maciejewski PK, Maercker A, Boelen PA, Prigerson HG: "Prolonged grief disorder" and "persistent complex bereavement disorder," but not "complicated grief," are one and the same diagnostic entity: an analysis of data from the Yale Bereavement Study. World Psychiatry 15(3):266–275, 2016 27717273

Maciejewski PK, Falzarano FB, She WJ, et al: A micro-sociological theory of adjustment to loss. Curr Opin Psychol 43:96–101, 2022 34333375

Maercker A, Brewin CR, Bryant RA et al: Diagnosis and classification of disorders specifically associated with stress: proposals for ICD-11. World Psychiatry 12(3):198–206, 2013 24096776

Parkes CM: Bereavement and mental illness, 1: a clinical study of the grief of bereaved psychiatric patients. Br J Med Psychol 38:1–12, 1965a 14300775

Parkes CM: Bereavement and mental illness, 2: a classification of bereavement reactions. Br J Med Psychol 38:13–26, 1965b 14300774

Parkes C: Bereavement: Studies of Grief in Adult Life. London, Tavistock, 1972

Parkes CM: Bereavement in adult life. BMJ 316(7134):856–859, 1998 9549464

Parkes CM, Weiss RS: Recovery From Bereavement. New York, Basic Books, 1983

Prigerson HG, Jacobs S: Traumatic grief as a distinct disorder: a rationale, consensus criteria, and a preliminary empirical test, in Handbook of Bereavement Research: Consequences, Coping, and Care. Edited by Stroebe MS, Hansson RO, Stroebe W, Schut H. Washington, DC, American Psychological Association, 2001, pp 613–645

Prigerson HG, Maciejewski PK: Prolonged Grief Disorder (PG-13) Scale. Available at: https://endoflife.weill.cornell.edu/advanced-directives/pg-13-self-report-wcm. Accessed March 23, 2023.

Prigerson HG, Frank E, Kasl SV, et al: Complicated grief and bereavement-related depression as distinct disorders: preliminary empirical validation in elderly bereaved spouses. Am J Psychiatry 152(1):22–30, 1995a 7802116

Prigerson HG, Maciejewski PK, Reynolds CF III, et al: Inventory of complicated grief: a scale to measure maladaptive symptoms of loss. Psychiatry Res 59(1–2):65–79, 1995b 8771222

Prigerson HG, Bierhals AJ, Kasl SV, et al: Complicated grief as a disorder distinct from bereavement-related depression and anxiety: a replication study. Am J Psychiatry 153(11):1484–1486, 1996 8890686

Prigerson HG, Bierhals AJ, Kasl SV, et al: Traumatic grief as a risk factor for mental and physical morbidity. Am J Psychiatry 154(5):616–623, 1997 9137115

Prigerson HG, Shear MK, Jacobs SC, et al: Consensus criteria for traumatic grief: a preliminary empirical test. Br J Psychiatry 174:67–73, 1999 10211154

Prigerson HG, Horowitz MJ, Jacobs SC, et al: Prolonged grief disorder: psychometric validation of criteria proposed for DSM-V and ICD-11. PLoS Med 6(8):e1000121, 2009 19652695

Prigerson HG, Boelen PA, Xu J, et al: Validation of the new DSM-5-TR criteria for prolonged grief disorder and the PG-13-Revised (PG-13-R) scale. World Psychiatry 20(1):96–106, 2021a 33432758

Prigerson HG, Kakarala S, Gang J, Maciejewski PK: History and status of prolonged grief disorder as a psychiatric diagnosis. Annu Rev Clin Psychol 17:109–126, 2021b 33524263

Regier DA, Kuhl EA, Kupfer DJ: The DSM-5: classification and criteria changes. World Psychiatry 12(2):92–98, 2013 23737408

Reynolds CF III, Frank E, Perel JM, et al: Nortriptyline and interpersonal psychotherapy as maintenance therapies for recurrent major depression: a randomized controlled trial in patients older than 59 years. JAMA 281(1):39–45, 1999 9892449

Shear K, Frank E, Houck PR, Reynolds CF III: Treatment of complicated grief: a randomized controlled trial. JAMA 293(21):2601–2608, 2005 15928281

Stelzer E-M, Zhou N, Maercker A, et al: Prolonged grief disorder and the cultural crisis. Front Psychol 10:2982, 2020 31998204

World Health Organization: International Classification of Diseases, 11th Revision. Geneva, World Health Organization, 2022

Clinically Relevant Correlates of Prolonged Grief Disorder

Paul K. Maciejewski, Ph.D.
Holly G. Prigerson, Ph.D.

PGD is conceptually and diagnostically distinct from other psychiatric disorders. That said, several psychological, psychiatric, and behavioral and physical health correlates of PGD are prominent, significant, and clinically relevant, which we describe in this chapter.

Foremost, it is important to acknowledge that PGD is associated with substantial co-occurring psychiatric morbidity. In a meta-analysis (Heeke et al. 2019) of correlates of PGD among adults exposed to violent loss, including 37 studies published between 2003 and 2017, PGD was shown to be highly comorbid with major depressive disorder (MDD) ($r=0.57$), generalized anxiety disorder (GAD) ($r=0.52$), and PTSD ($r=0.59$). PGD was also found to be closely associated with suicidality ($r=0.41$) and rumination about the loss ($r=0.42$) (Heeke et al. 2019). Although the meta-analysis was restricted to studies of bereaved individuals exposed to violent loss, these correlates of PGD are consistent with correlates observed in more general bereaved populations. Here we take a closer look at the primary clinically relevant correlates of PGD that have emerged in the literature.

Rumination: A Transdiagnostic Risk for Psychopathology

Although it may not be the most clinically troubling psychological correlate of PGD, we begin with rumination because it is associated not only with PGD but also with other clinically relevant correlates of PGD. As illustrated in Figure 5–1, rumination is associated with prolonged grief, depression and anxiety, suicidality, and perception of stressful life events. Thus, rumination as a correlate may also provide insight into other clinically relevant correlates of PGD.

We examine more closely the connection between rumination and prolonged grief later in this chapter. Here we elaborate on the concept of rumination and its links to other salient clinical features associated with PGD, such as comorbid psychopathology and suicidality.

Rumination is a repetitive thought process in which an individual incessantly dwells on past events and present predicaments. One may view rumination as a self-focused preoccupation with perceived missteps, mistakes, misfortunes, insults, losses, and missed opportunities. Rumination is often coupled with feelings of regret, anger, guilt, and envy. Rumination may be reflective or brooding. Whereas *reflective rumination* is typically a nonjudgmental, purposeful turning inward to engage in cognitive problem-solving, *brooding rumination* is typically an idle, negative comparison of one's present situation with some unmet standard (Treynor et al. 2003).

Susan Nolen-Hoeksema and her colleagues conducted extensive research on rumination and its role in the onset and maintenance of psychopathology. She initially considered the role that rumination plays in mental health somewhat narrowly, as a repetitive thought-process mechanism by which depressed individuals prolong their depressive episodes (Nolen-Hoeksema 1991). In this context, within Nolen-Hoeksema's response styles theory of the duration of depression, rumination is a cognitive response to depression in which one's symptoms and possible causes and consequences of one's symptoms of depression become the objects of one's rumination. According to Nolen-Hoeksema, ruminative responses to depression "prolong depression because they allow the depressed mood to negatively bias thinking and interfere with instrumental behavior and problem-solving" (Nolen-Hoeksema 1991). Although Nolen-Hoeksema and colleagues eventually revised these initial theories (Nolen-Hoeksema et al. 2008; Treynor et al. 2003), the notion that rumination prolongs negative affect may have some bearing on understanding cognitive mechanisms by which grief may

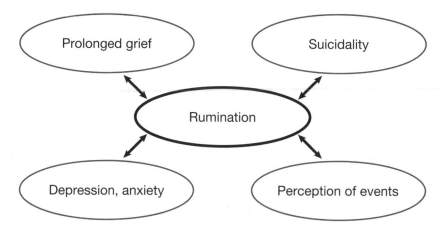

Figure 5–1. Hypothesized centrality of rumination in the onset and maintenance of psychopathology in bereavement.

be prolonged. Preoccupation with thoughts or memories of a deceased person is a core symptom of PGD and in many instances may be viewed as a form of rumination. Consistent with Nolen-Hoeksema's theory that rumination prolongs depression, ruminative preoccupation with thoughts of the decedent may serve (in a mechanistic sense) to perpetuate and prolong a bereft individual's grief. It is worth noting that, in contrast with depression, PGD-related ruminations may have a bittersweet flavor to them, providing comfort of the rewarding connection to the deceased person, tinged with sorrow over missing this connection.

Nolen-Hoeksema and colleagues, supported by evidence, ultimately began to view rumination as a maladaptive cognitive emotion-regulation strategy that impacts the onset or course of depression and other psychiatric syndromes transdiagnostically (Aldao and Nolen-Hoeksema 2010; Aldao et al. 2010; McLaughlin and Nolen-Hoeksema 2011). In particular, rumination plays a prominent role in the etiology and comorbidity of depression and anxiety, and particularly in the intrusive thoughts characteristic of PTSD (McLaughlin and Nolen-Hoeksema 2011). The studies supporting these conclusions about rumination as a transdiagnostic factor associated with the development of multiple types of psychopathology neither focused on bereavement nor included assessments of prolonged grief (which, at that time, was not officially recognized as a form of psychopathology). Rumination may also play a role in the etiology of prolonged grief and perhaps explain its comorbidities with depression, anxiety, and emotional trauma.

Rumination regulates not only various forms of psychopathology (e.g., depression and anxiety) but also a specific symptom of intense emotional pain: anger. If related to the death of a close other, anger is also a symptom of PGD. Rusting and Nolen-Hoeksema (1998) found that rumination amplified anger, that women were more likely to distract themselves than ruminate when they were angry, and that men were equally likely to distract themselves or ruminate when they were angry. Thus, it is likely that rumination exacerbates loss-related emotional pain of bereft individuals. It is also plausible that, because women tend to not ruminate when they are angry, anger related to the death of a close other may be, because of a sex difference in rumination in response to anger, particularly painful for men.

Rumination plays a significant role in relationships between stressful life events and internalized psychopathology. Nolen-Hoeksema and colleagues found that rumination mediates effects of stressful life events on anxiety in adolescents and both anxiety and depression in adults (Michl et al. 2013). Rumination about stressful life events may capture and perpetuate psychological distress associated with those events and, thereby, sustain or precipitate depression and anxiety. The notion that rumination about past events serves to preserve those events (as well as related memories and emotions) may have important implications for understanding the role of rumination in the etiology of PGD. For example, incessant repetitive thought (i.e., rumination) about the decedent (or the circumstances of the death) may serve to trap the bereft individual's experience of the loss in an (atemporal) infinite loop, perpetuating the psychological distress (and response) associated with the loss and thereby prolonging grief.

Both brooding and reflection, the two dimensions of rumination, predict suicidal ideation, which is strongly associated with PGD. In a community sample of adults ($N=1,134$), Miranda and Nolen-Hoeksema (2007) found that brooding and reflective pondering assessed at baseline independently predicted suicidal ideation at 1-year follow-up, adjusting for baseline suicidal ideation. Further, they found that depression mediated the effect of brooding on suicidal ideation but did not mediate the effect of reflection on suicidal ideation. In bereavement, PGD predicts suicidal ideation independently of depression. The possibility that reflective, as opposed to brooding (depressive), rumination leads to greater suicidal ideation among individuals with PGD warrants further consideration.

Finally, although rumination is most often considered a mechanism by which repetitive thoughts sustain or augment negative affect, it also blocks other, more adaptive, cognitive and behavioral mechanisms for regulating emotions. For example, rumination is associated with cognitive inflexibility

(Davis and Nolen-Hoeksema 2000) and negative autobiographical memories (Lyubomirsky et al. 1998) and may interfere with instrumental behavior and problem-solving approaches to emotion regulation (Nolen-Hoeksema 1991). Thus, cognitive-behavioral therapies for PGD need to confront and address rumination.

Rumination, Worry, and Avoidance

Once PGD was on a path to be included as a new syndrome in ICD-11 and DSM-5, Maarten Eisma and colleagues published a series of reports examining negative repetitive thoughts in the context of bereavement and in relation to prolonged grief symptom severity (Eisma et al. 2013, 2015a, 2015b, 2017, 2020). These investigations examined not only *rumination* (negative repetitive thoughts about past events and present predicaments) but *worry* (negative repetitive thoughts about uncertain future events) as well, in relation to prolonged grief. They also examined various *avoidance* processes (e.g., suppression, memory/experiential avoidance, behavioral avoidance, and loss-related avoidance) as mediators of the effects of rumination and worry in bereavement on prolonged grief and depression.

In a longitudinal study of avoidance processes in bereft individuals as mediators of relationships between rumination and severity of grief and depressive symptoms, Eisma et al. (2013) found that, controlling for symptom severity at baseline, *experiential avoidance* (assessed at 6 months) mediated the effect of baseline rumination on subsequent grief severity (assessed at 12 months), and *experiential avoidance* and *behavioral avoidance* mediated the effect of rumination on subsequent depression. They also found evidence that suppression may mediate the effect of rumination on subsequent grief severity, but not subsequent depression severity. Thus, rumination in bereavement augments and perpetuates grief and depression through one common avoidance mechanism (experiential avoidance for both grief and depression) and two distinct avoidance mechanisms (suppression for grief and behavioral avoidance for depression).

In a longitudinal study of effects of subtypes of *depressive rumination* (brooding and reflection) and *grief rumination* (rumination about injustice, meaning, reactions, relationships, and counterfactual thinking) on concurrent and subsequent severity of grief and depression in bereft individuals, Eisma et al. (2015b) found that, overall, grief rumination as opposed to depressive rumination explained more variance in both grief and depression symptom severity. Grief rumination about injustice predicted higher grief severity both concurrently and prospectively and higher depression severity prospectively. Grief rumination about emotional reactions predicted lower grief severity prospectively. Reflective depressive rumination predicted reductions in both grief and depressive symptom severity prospectively. Thus, grief rumination about injustice, perhaps associated with emotions of anger and bitterness, may be particularly fierce in stoking and prolonging grief and precipitating depression, whereas other types of rumination—rumination about emotional reactions and reflection—may in time reduce grief and depression symptom severity. These effects may prove relevant to interventions for individuals bereaved because of human misdeeds or violence, as in the case of war and other atrocities.

Using an avoidance task to assess autonomic behavior tendencies, Eisma et al. (2015a) investigated associations between rumination and implicit loss avoidance among bereft individuals. Participants used a joystick to push away from or pull toward themselves paired image/word stimuli representing their loss, ambiguously representing loss, and not representing loss. The results showed that greater rumination was associated with participants' being faster in pushing loss stimuli away from themselves and slower in pulling loss stimuli toward themselves, indicating that rumination is associated with implicit loss avoidance. Importantly, this observed effect of rumination on implicit loss avoidance remained significant when controlling for depressive or posttraumatic stress symptom levels, but not when controlling for prolonged grief symptom levels. Thus, this effect of rumination on implicit loss avoidance appears to be independent of depression and posttraumatic stress but confounded with prolonged grief.

After determining that worry was concurrently associated with and prospectively predictive of higher levels of anxiety, depression, and prolonged grief among bereft individuals, Eisma et al. (2017) sought to determine whether effects of worry on levels of grief and depression in bereavement are independent of effects of rumination on these outcomes; they also studied the extent to which *loss-related avoidance* and behavioral avoidance of activities mediate the effects of rumination and worry on grief and depression (Eisma et al. 2020). In a cross-sectional study of bereft individuals ($N=474$), they found that rumination and worry were independently associated with higher levels of both depression and prolonged grief symptoms. They also found that loss-related avoidance and behavioral avoidance of activities partially mediated associations of rumination and worry with prolonged grief symptoms, whereas behavioral avoidance of activities alone only partially mediated associations of rumination and worry with depression symptoms. Thus, worry and rumination appear to be distinct, independent mechanisms that exacerbate grief and depression in bereavement.

Further, whereas behavioral avoidance of activities appears to play a role in these mechanisms for both prolonged grief and depression, loss-related avoidance plays a role in these mechanisms only for prolonged grief alone.

Comorbid Psychopathology

It is common for bereavement-related mental disorders to co-occur with PGD. Indeed, PGD has been recognized as a psychiatric syndrome in part because it has been shown to be distinct from other established "nearest neighbor" syndromes such as depression, anxiety, and PTSD. For example, in a recent study (Prigerson et al. 2021) analyzing three independent bereaved samples from prospective studies of PGD conducted in the United States, the United Kingdom, and the Netherlands, meeting DSM-5-TR criteria for PGD was associated with meeting criteria for other mental disorders (MDD, $\phi=0.25$; GAD, $\phi=0.26$; PTSD, $\phi=0.12$) and severity of symptoms of depression and PTSD both concurrently and prospectively. Thus, MDD, GAD, and PTSD are often comorbid with PGD, though perhaps not as comorbid in community-based bereaved samples as clinicians might expect.

It is instructive to view psychiatric syndromes with heterogeneous symptomatology (as in the case of syndromes that present as an amalgam of comorbid disorders) from a dimensional as opposed to a categorical perspective. Rather than seeing a person as having multiple, distinct, comorbid disorders, it may be more helpful to see that person as having a single syndrome that has features associated with each of several distinct disorders. Latent class analysis (LCA) is a methodological research tool that can be used to identify coherent syndromes that display features of multiple distinct disorders.

Paul Boelen and colleagues have used LCA in several studies of comorbid psychopathology in bereft individuals, focusing on symptoms of prolonged grief, depression, and posttraumatic stress; in each study, they defined three classes of grief. Assessing symptoms of PGD, PTSD, and MDD in a Dutch community sample of bereft individuals ($N=496$), Djelantik et al. (2017) defined, using LCA, a resilient class, a PGD class, and a combined PGD/PTSD class. In a study using LCA of patterns of PGD, PTSD, and MDD symptoms in bereft individuals ($N=322$), Boelen and Lenferink (2020) described the three groups as a low-symptom class (35.4%), a predominantly PGD class (29.8%), and a high-symptom class (34.8%), members of which had symptoms associated with all three disorders. These studies suggest that PGD is equally likely to be present in one of two forms, either an almost pure form (i.e., with few features associated with other disorders) or a highly comorbid form (with features of PTSD and MDD).

Boelen and colleagues reported similar results using LCA in more narrowly defined bereft populations. In a study using LCA of symptoms of PGD and MDD in a sample of individuals bereft because of an unnatural death (accident, suicide, homicide, etc.; $N=425$) (Boelen et al. 2016), the groups were a resilient class (25.3%), a predominantly PGD class (39.2%), and a combined PGD/MDD class (35.5%). In a study using LCA of symptoms of PGD, MDD, and PTSD in individuals bereaved by the 2014 MH17 plane crash in Ukraine ($N=167$) (Lenferink et al. 2017), the three groups were a resilient class (20.0%) characterized by low probability of PGD, MDD, and PTSD symptom clusters; a PGD class (41.8%) characterized by moderate to high probability of PGD; and a combined class (38.2%) characterized by moderate to high probability of PGD, MDD, and PTSD symptom clusters. The latter two LCA studies of individuals bereft by unnatural deaths suggest again that PGD is equally likely to present in one of two forms, pure PGD or PGD that is highly comorbid with MDD or PTSD.

Suicidal Thoughts and Behaviors

Bereft individuals' ruminations and reflections on the lives and deaths of close others often lead them to examine existential questions and confront their own mortality. For bereft individuals with PGD, these thought processes may incorporate a sense of futility about the future (Prigerson et al. 1999b) and ultimately result in suicidal thoughts and behaviors in adults (Prigerson et al. 1997; Szanto et al. 2006), as well as suicidal ideation in children and adolescents (Melhem et al. 2007) and older adults (Szanto et al. 1997). Indeed, for bereft individuals with PGD, these ruminations and reflections may be accompanied by a sense of confusion about one's role in life or loss of identity (one symptom of PGD), coupled with a sense that life is meaningless without the person who died (another symptom of PGD) and a feeling of being alone or lonely (a sign of social-emotional isolation) without the deceased (yet another symptom of PGD). Further, as noted earlier, rumination, a cognitive correlate of prolonged grief (Heeke et al. 2019), is predictive of future suicidal ideation independent of present suicidal ideation (Miranda and Nolen-Hoeksema 2007). Thus, it is unsurprising that suicidal thoughts and behaviors are strongly and unambiguously associated with PGD (Heeke et al. 2019; Prigerson et al. 1999a, 2021).

Bereaved individuals are at heightened risk of suicidal thoughts (Stroebe et al. 2005) and suicide (Guldin et al. 2015). Bereaved subgroups, such as those who meet criteria for PGD and those bereaved by suicide, have an even greater risk of suicidal ideation and attempted suicide (Garssen et al.

2011; Pitman 2018; Prigerson et al. 1999a, 2021). Bereaved persons who meet diagnostic criteria for PGD are three to five times more likely to engage in suicidal thinking than those who do not meet criteria (Latham and Prigerson 2004; Lichtenthal et al. 2011; Prigerson et al. 1999a). A stunning national survey in the United Kingdom found that 9% of those bereaved by suicide subsequently made a suicide attempt (Pitman et al. 2016). Furthermore, not only are those who meet criteria for PGD and those bereaved by suicide at elevated risk for suicidal thoughts and behaviors, but they are also less likely to receive informal support or access mental health care (Lichtenthal et al. 2011; Pitman et al. 2017).

It is worth noting that, although suicidal thoughts and behaviors are often associated with depression, prolonged grief is a unique predictor of suicidal thoughts and behaviors in bereavement, independent of the effects of depression. Prigerson et al. (1999a) found that adults bereft by suicide who met (as opposed to those who did not meet) criteria for traumatic grief (a predecessor of PGD) were four times more likely to engage in suicidal ideation, controlling for depression. In another study of adults bereft by suicide, Mitchell et al. (2005) found that those who met (as opposed to those who did not meet) criteria for complicated grief (another predecessor of PGD) were nine times more likely to engage in suicidal ideation, after controlling for depression. In a study of help-seeking individuals who met criteria for complicated grief, Szanto et al. (2006) found in a multiple logistic regression analysis that only the severity of complicated grief symptoms and history of a suicide attempt, and neither severity of depressive symptoms nor lifetime major depressive disorder, were significantly associated with postloss suicidal behavior. It appears reasonable to conclude from these studies that extreme symptoms of PGD pose significant risks for suicidal thoughts and behaviors, and that these risks are greater than and independent of those posed by symptoms of bereavement-related depression and anxiety.

Substance Abuse

Yearning, the most characteristic, defining symptom of grief and PGD, has some similarity with *craving*, a core symptom of addictive disorders. This similarity between yearning and craving suggests that neurobiological correlates of PGD may overlap with those of addictive disorders. In an event-related functional-MRI investigation of neurobiological correlates of complicated grief (CG; a predecessor of PGD) and yearning in a sample of bereaved women (11 CG and 12 non-CG), O'Connor et al. (2008) found that whereas both CG and non-CG participants displayed pain-related neural activity in response to reminders of the deceased, only those with CG displayed re-ward-related activity in the nucleus accumbens. Activity in this neurobiolog-ical reward center was also positively correlated with self-reported yearning for the decedent, suggesting that yearning may be, in essence, "craving love." It is important to highlight that the yearning and reward activation was spe-cific to images of the deceased loved one. In a broader systematic review of research relating neurobiological reward systems to PGD, Kakarala et al. (2020) found further nascent evidence that reward systems play a role in the onset and maintenance of PGD symptoms. Thus, there may be a common neurobiological basis for yearning and addictive behaviors.

In a systematic review of research on the relationship between substance misuse and complicated grief, Parisi et al. (2019) found evidence of a posi-tive bidirectional relationship between complicated grief and substance misuse. That is, on the one hand, individuals with substance misuse were at increased risk for subsequent development of complicated grief, and on the other hand, complicated grief predicted increases in smoking and alcohol dependence. These findings appear to be consistent with the notion that PGD and addictive behaviors have some common denominator. Although Parisi et al. highlighted evidence in support of relationships between disor-dered grief and smoking and alcohol dependence, studies in their system-atic review also suggest that disordered grief may be related to substance use disorders (SUDs) more broadly. Masferrer et al. (2017) reported that bereft individuals with SUDs (i.e., alcohol, heroin, and cocaine dependence) were more likely to meet criteria for complicated grief than those without SUDs, and, in another study, that >80% of drug-dependent patients increased drug consumption after suffering the loss of a close other (Masferrer et al. 2015). Prigerson et al. (1997) also found that bereaved participants who were clas-sified as having what we now term PGD were >16 times more likely to re-port increases in smoking than those without PGD.

Mortality and Physical Health

This chapter has focused primarily on clinically relevant psychological and behavioral correlates of PGD. However, bereavement generally and PGD specifically have noteworthy, clinically relevant associations with mortality and physical health. DSM-5-TR criteria for PGD, as well as criteria for other disorders, require that the syndrome is associated with significant func-tional impairment that may include physical dysfunction. It is worth noting that meeting the symptom criterion for PGD alone, without including the so-called impairment criterion, is significantly related to functional disability and poor quality of life (Prigerson et al. 2009).

Studies have found that individuals bereft by the death of a spouse (widowers and widows), compared with married individuals, have higher rates of death. Parkes et al. (1969) found that, within the first 6 months of bereavement, the rate at which widowers died was 40% greater than for married men of the same age. Furthermore, they found that this higher rate of mortality in close proximity to the death of a spouse was largely because of widowers dying from coronary thrombosis and other arteriosclerotic and degenerative heart disease, supporting their suggestion that some widowers may die from having a "broken heart." Consistent with these conclusions, a study of determinants of myocardial infarction onset found that the incidence rate of acute myocardial infarction onset was significantly elevated 20-fold within 1 day of the death of a significant person (not only a spouse) and declined steadily on each subsequent day (Mostofsky et al. 2012). In a large-scale longitudinal cohort study of the effect of widowhood on mortality by the causes of death of both spouses in a nationally representative sample of elderly married couples in the United States followed from 1993 to 2002 (N=373,189), Elwert and Christakis (2008) found that, for both men and women, the death of a spouse from any cause increased the survivor's cause-specific mortality for almost all causes, including cancers, infections, and cardiovascular diseases, to varying degrees; they concluded that the effect of widowhood on mortality is not restricted to one aspect of human biology. Intriguingly, Prigerson et al. (1997) found that widows and widowers who, 6 months after the loss, met (as opposed to those who did not meet) criteria for traumatic grief had higher rates of heart trouble and cancer 6–25 months after the loss. Thus, it is plausible that PGD plays some role in bereavement-related risk for mortality.

Toblin et al. (2012) investigated relationships between grief and physical health outcomes in a sample of U.S. soldiers returning from combat in Iraq or Afghanistan (N=1,522). One in five of these soldiers reported difficulty coping with grief over the death of someone close. Controlling for demographic characteristics, combat experiences, injuries, PTSD, depression, and other factors, Toblin et al. found that difficulty coping with grief was significantly related to soldiers' high somatic symptom scores (including assessments of pain, dizziness, heart pounding or racing, shortness of breath, nausea, fatigue, and sleep problems), poor general health, missed work, medical service utilization, difficulty carrying a heavy load, and difficulty performing physical training. These findings suggest that severe grief has a detrimental impact on a broad swath of physical and occupational health outcomes.

The idea that grief—a social-psychological experience—has an impact on biological processes (physical health) needs some explanation. Berkman (1995) noted that people who are socially isolated are at heightened risk of death, that supportive social relationships must provide a sense of belonging and intimacy and promote competency and self-efficacy to promote physical health, and that social support must somehow be related to more direct physiologic pathways that undergird physical health, e.g., biological mechanisms that support neuroendocrine or immunologic function. To the latter point, in a review of research on physiological processes potentially underlying links between social support and disease outcomes, Uchino (2006) found that social support appears to be related to more positive "biological profiles" across disease-relevant systems (e.g., cardiovascular, neuroendocrine, and immune). Furthermore, and relatedly, in connection with the detrimental effects of social isolation on physical health, Steptoe et al. (2004) have found that *loneliness* (a symptom of PGD) appears to have adverse effects on biological stress processes relevant to physical health (i.e., neuroendocrine, cardiovascular, inflammatory) and that relationships between loneliness and stress-related inflammatory and neuroendocrine responses are more pronounced in women (Hackett et al. 2012). Thus, is it plausible that relationships between PGD and poor physical health may be explained by these pathways; these conjectures have yet to be empirically confirmed. Research is needed to determine associations between bereavement, psychological responses such as grief and PGD, and physical health outcomes that heighten risk of death in mourners.

References

Aldao A, Nolen-Hoeksema S: Specificity of cognitive emotion regulation strategies: a transdiagnostic examination. Behav Res Ther 48(10):974–983, 2010 20591413

Aldao A, Nolen-Hoeksema S, Schweizer S: Emotion-regulation strategies across psychopathology: a meta-analytic review. Clin Psychol Rev 30(2):217–237, 2010 20015584

Berkman LF: The role of social relations in health promotion. Psychosom Med 57(3):245–254, 1995 7652125

Boelen PA, Lenferink LIM: Symptoms of prolonged grief, posttraumatic stress, and depression in recently bereaved people: symptom profiles, predictive value, and cognitive behavioural correlates. Soc Psychiatry Psychiatr Epidemiol 55(6):765–777, 2020 31535165

Boelen PA, Reijntjes A, Djelantik AAAMJ, Smid GE: Prolonged grief and depression after unnatural loss: latent class analyses and cognitive correlates. Psychiatry Res 30;240:358–363, 2016 27138832

Davis RN, Nolen-Hoeksema S: Cognitive inflexibility among ruminators and non-ruminators. Cognit Ther Res 24(6):699–711, 2000

Djelantik AAAMJ, Smid GE, Kleber RJ, Boelen PA: Symptoms of prolonged grief, post-traumatic stress, and depression after loss in a Dutch community sample: a latent class analysis. Psychiatry Res 247:276–281, 2017 27936439

Eisma MC, Stroebe MS, Schut HAW, et al: Avoidance processes mediate the relationship between rumination and symptoms of complicated grief and depression following loss. J Abnorm Psychol 122(4):961–970, 2013 24364599

Eisma MC, Rinck M, Stroebe MS, et al: Rumination and implicit avoidance following bereavement: an approach avoidance task investigation. J Behav Ther Exp Psychiatry 47:84–91, 2015a 25499772

Eisma MC, Schut HAW, Stroebe MS, et al: Adaptive and maladaptive rumination after loss: a three-wave longitudinal study. Br J Clin Psychol 54(2):163–180, 2015b 25229192

Eisma MC, Boelen PA, Schut HAW, Stroebe MS: Does worry affect adjustment to bereavement? A longitudinal investigation. Anxiety Stress Coping 30(3):243–252, 2017 27575924

Eisma MC, de Lang TA, Boelen PA: How thinking hurts: rumination, worry, and avoidance processes in adjustment to bereavement. Clin Psychol Psychother 27(4):548–558, 2020 32103569

Elwert F, Christakis NA: The effect of widowhood on mortality by the causes of death of both spouses. Am J Public Health 98(11):2092–2098, 2008 18511733

Garssen J, Deerenberg I, Mackenbach JP, et al: Familial risk of early suicide: variations by age and sex of children and parents. Suicide Life Threat Behav 41:585–593, 2011 21815914

Guldin MB, Li J, Pedersen HS, et al: Incidence of suicide among persons who had a parent who died during their childhood: a population-based cohort study. JAMA Psychiatry 72(12):1227–1234, 2015 26558351

Hackett RA, Hamer M, Endrighi R, et al: Loneliness and stress-related inflammatory and neuroendocrine responses in older men and women. Psychoneuroendocrinology 37(11):1801–1809, 2012 22503139

Heeke C, Kampisiou C, Niemeyer H, Knaevelsrud C: A systematic review and meta-analysis of correlates of prolonged grief disorder in adults exposed to violent loss. Eur J Psychotraumatol 10(1):1583524, 2019 30949303

Kakarala SE, Roberts KE, Rogers M, et al: The neurobiological reward system in Prolonged Grief Disorder (PGD): a systematic review. Psychiatry Res Neuroimaging 303:111135, 2020 32629197

Latham AE, Prigerson HG: Suicidality and bereavement: complicated grief as psychiatric disorder presenting greatest risk for suicidality. Suicide Life Threat Behav 34(4):350–362, 2004 15585457

Lenferink LIM, de Keijser J, Smid GE, et al: Prolonged grief, depression, and post-traumatic stress in disaster-bereaved individuals: latent class analysis. Eur J Psychotraumatol 8(1):1298311, 2017 28451067

Lichtenthal WG, Nilsson M, Kissane DW, et al: Underutilization of mental health services among bereaved caregivers with prolonged grief disorder. Psychiatr Serv 62(10):1225–1229, 2011 21969652

Lyubomirsky S, Caldwell ND, Nolen-Hoeksema S: Effects of ruminative and distracting responses to depressed mood on retrieval of autobiographical memories. J Pers Soc Psychol 75(1):166–177, 1998 9686457

Masferrer L, Garre-Olmo J, Caparros B: Is there any relationship between drug users' bereavement and substance consumption? Heroin Addict Relat Clin Probl 17(6):23–30, 2015

Masferrer L, Garre-Olmo J, Caparrós B: Is complicated grief a risk factor for substance use? A comparison of substance-users and normative grievers. Addict Res Theory 25(5):361–367, 2017

McLaughlin KA, Nolen-Hoeksema S: Rumination as a transdiagnostic factor in depression and anxiety. Behav Res Ther 49(3):186–193, 2011 21238951

Melhem NM, Moritz G, Walker M, et al: Phenomenology and correlates of complicated grief in children and adolescents. J Am Acad Child Adolesc Psychiatry 46(4):493–499, 2007 17420684

Michl LC, McLaughlin KA, Shepherd K, Nolen-Hoeksema S: Rumination as a mechanism linking stressful life events to symptoms of depression and anxiety: longitudinal evidence in early adolescents and adults. J Abnorm Psychol 122(2):339–352, 2013 23713497

Miranda R, Nolen-Hoeksema S: Brooding and reflection: rumination predicts suicidal ideation at one-year follow-up in a community sample. Behav Res Ther 45(12):3088–3095, 2007 17825248

Mitchell AM, Kim Y, Prigerson HG, Mortimer MK: Complicated grief and suicidal ideation in adult survivors of suicide. Suicide Life Threat Behav 35(5):498–506, 2005 16268767

Mostofsky E, Maclure M, Sherwood JB, et al: Risk of acute myocardial infarction after the death of a significant person in one's life: the Determinants of Myocardial Infarction Onset Study. Circulation 125(3):491–496, 2012 22230481

Nolen-Hoeksema S: Responses to depression and their effects on the duration of depressive episodes. J Abnorm Psychol 100(4):569–582, 1991 1757671

Nolen-Hoeksema S, Wisco BE, Lyubomirsky S: Rethinking rumination. Perspect Psychol Sci 3(5):400–424, 2008 26158958

O'Connor MF, Wellisch DK, Stanton AL, et al: Craving love? Enduring grief activates brain's reward center. Neuroimage 42(2):969–972, 2008 18559294

Parisi A, Sharma A, Howard MO, Blank Wilson A: The relationship between substance misuse and complicated grief: a systematic review. J Subst Abuse Treat 103:43–57, 2019 31229191

Parkes CM, Benjamin B, Fitzgerald RG: Broken heart: a statistical study of increased mortality among widowers. Br Med J 1(5646):740–743, 1969 5769860

Pitman A: Addressing suicide risk in partners and relatives bereaved by suicide. Br J Psychiatry 212(4):197–198, 2018 29557756

Pitman AL, Osborn DPJ, Rantell K, King MB: Bereavement by suicide as a risk factor for suicide attempt: a cross-sectional national UK-wide study of 3432 young bereaved adults. BMJ Open 6(1):e009948, 2016 26813968

Pitman AL, Rantell K, Moran P, et al: Support received after bereavement by suicide and other sudden deaths: a cross-sectional UK study of 3432 young bereaved adults. BMJ Open 7(5):e014487, 2017 28554915

Prigerson HG, Bierhals AJ, Kasl SV, et al: Traumatic grief as a risk factor for mental and physical morbidity. Am J Psychiatry 154(5):616–623, 1997 9137115

Prigerson HG, Bridge J, Maciejewski PK, et al: Influence of traumatic grief on suicidal ideation among young adults. Am J Psychiatry 156(12):1994–1995, 1999a 10588419

Prigerson HG, Shear MK, Jacobs SC, et al: Consensus criteria for traumatic grief. A preliminary empirical test. Br J Psychiatry 174:67–73, 1999b 10211154

Prigerson HG, Horowitz MJ, Jacobs SC, et al: Prolonged grief disorder: psychometric validation of criteria proposed for DSM-V and ICD-11. PLoS Med 6(8):e1000121, 2009 19652695

Prigerson HG, Boelen PA, Xu J, et al: Validation of the new DSM-5-TR criteria for prolonged grief disorder and the PG-13-Revised (PG-13-R) scale. World Psychiatry 20(1):96–106, 2021 33432758

Rusting CL, Nolen-Hoeksema S: Regulating responses to anger: effects of rumination and distraction on angry mood. J Pers Soc Psychol 74(3):790–803, 1998 9523420

Steptoe A, Owen N, Kunz-Ebrecht SR, Brydon L: Loneliness and neuroendocrine, cardiovascular, and inflammatory stress responses in middle-aged men and women. Psychoneuroendocrinology 29(5):593–611, 2004 15041083

Stroebe M, Stroebe W, Abakoumkin G: The broken heart: suicidal ideation in bereavement. Am J Psychiatry 162(11):2178–2180, 2005 16263862

Szanto K, Prigerson H, Houck P, et al: Suicidal ideation in elderly bereaved: the role of complicated grief. Suicide Life Threat Behav 27(2):194–207, 1997 9260302

Szanto K, Shear MK, Houck PR, et al: Indirect self-destructive behavior and overt suicidality in patients with complicated grief. J Clin Psychiatry 67(2):233–239, 2006 16566618

Toblin RL, Riviere LA, Thomas JL, et al: Grief and physical health outcomes in U.S. soldiers returning from combat. J Affect Disord 136(3):469–475, 2012 22154707

Treynor W, Gonzalez R, Nolen-Hoeksema S: Rumination reconsidered: a psychometric analysis. Cognit Ther Res 27(3):247–259, 2003

Uchino BN: Social support and health: a review of physiological processes potentially underlying links to disease outcomes. J Behav Med 29(4):377–387, 2006 16758315

6

Epidemiology of Prolonged Grief Disorder

Paul K. Maciejewski, Ph.D.
Holly G. Prigerson, Ph.D.

PGD is a newly recognized mental disorder. Because the criteria that define PGD have been settled only recently, information is limited regarding the prevalence, risk factors, protective factors, and possible risks of PGD based on DSM-5-TR (American Psychiatric Association 2022) and ICD-11 (World Health Organization 2022) assessments. In this chapter, we present a narrative review of the epidemiology of PGD as currently defined based on the latest data. Much of this evidence is from a variety of studies in countries across the globe; findings replicated in different cultural contexts are likely to be more generally valid.

Meeting the Bereavement Qualification for PGD

Bereavement is a necessary condition for a diagnosis of PGD. According to DSM-5-TR, an individual is a candidate for PGD only if bereaved by the death of a close other ≥12 months ago (for children and adolescents, ≥6 months ago). This necessary condition for PGD contains the operative term *bereaved*, qualifications about the time since the death, and the closeness of the relationship with the decedent.

The criterion for PGD is not simple bereavement. Simple bereavement—defined as a period of grief and mourning following the death of a close other—is a nearly universal human experience. At some point, virtually everyone survives the death of a dear relative or friend. For example, in 2019, ~3 million people died in the United States. Roughly 600,000 more died in 2020 than in 2019 (~3.6 million)[1] as COVID-19 became a leading cause of death (Woolf et al. 2021). Each decedent is survived by approximately nine close relatives (Verdery et al. 2020), and these survivors may be considered "simply" bereft by the decedent's death. Thus, ~30 million Americans, or up to 9% of the total U.S. population, are bereft by the death of a close relative (grandparent, parent, sibling, spouse, or child) each year. It is reasonable to assume that almost every adult in the United States has been bereft by the death of a close relative.

Having a close kinship is not the same as having a close interpersonal relationship with a decedent, of course. On the one hand, some individuals within a close kinship network (the nuclear family) may not have had close interpersonal relationships with the decedent—for instance, an absent or unknown parent—and, as a result, may be relatively unaffected by the death. On the other hand, an individual outside of the decedent's close kinship network—a close friend or partner—may have had a close interpersonal relationship with the decedent and be affected profoundly. Thus, it is not obvious which and how many individuals simply bereft by a decedent's death meet the bereavement criterion for PGD.

Death statistics provide insight into segments of the general population newly exposed to bereavement each year. Older-aged peers (spouses, siblings, cousins, and friends) and middle-aged adult progeny are likely to be bereft by deaths of older adults (age >65 years; ~74% of all deaths in the United States); middle-aged peers, younger-aged progeny, and older adult parents are likely to be bereft by deaths of middle-aged adults (ages 35–65; ~22% of all U.S. deaths); younger-aged peers and middle-aged parents are likely to be bereft by deaths of children, adolescents, and younger adults (age <35; ~4% of all U.S. deaths). Children, adolescents, and younger adults are most likely to be bereft by deaths of middle-aged parents.

A recent study (Rosner et al. 2021), designed to estimate prevalence of PGD in a representative sample of the general German population (N=2,498), provided information about the composition of a general bereft

---

[1] Preliminary U.S. death statistics show >3.6 million total deaths in 2020—at least 20% more deaths than in 2019 (usafacts.org).

population that would most likely meet the DSM-5-TR bereavement criterion for PGD. According to the study, only 36.6% of individuals in the total sample indicated that they had ever experienced the loss of a significant person: a substantial portion of the general population, but well below that which may have been expected to have ever experienced simple bereavement (the loss of a person within their close kinship network). In fact, counterintuitively, one in five widowed persons within the study sample reported that they had never experienced the loss of a significant person, highlighting the point that simple bereavement and having had a close kinship relationship to a person who has died are not sufficient for having had a close interpersonal relationship with the deceased. In the study, individuals who had lost a significant person were older (54.3 versus 44.7 years), more likely to be female (59.2% versus 49.7%), more likely to be widowed (17.3% versus 2.6%), and more likely to be retired (36.2% versus 17.0%) than those who had never lost a significant person. Thus, individuals within these demographic subgroups are more likely to meet the DSM-5-TR bereavement criterion for PGD and to be overrepresented in general population studies of bereavement.

The study in the general German population also provided loss-related information about the bereft (Rosner et al. 2021). Approximately two in five bereft individuals (40.9%) lost a parent. Given that this general bereft population was middle-aged on average, it was unsurprising that the most common significant loss was that of an older adult parent. Approximately one in five bereft individuals lost a partner (17.4%) or child (3.5%). Given that 17.3% of bereft individuals indicated that they were presently widowed (nearly the exact same proportion who indicated that their significant loss was that of a partner), loss of a spouse or partner is likely to be more significant to the bereft than most other losses. Again, given that the bereft population is middle-aged on average, loss of a child may often indicate loss of an adult child; loss of a child in childhood may be extremely rare. Other significant losses, among nearly two in five bereft individuals, included those of other family members (28.1%) or friends (9.6%). Overall, on average, losses occurred nearly 9 years before the survey was taken, indicating that bereft individuals endure and adapt to their losses over extended periods of time. Bereft individuals may be acutely affected by deaths of significant people in their lives for a few weeks or months, for many months or a few years, or even indefinitely.

Thus the death of an individual person precipitates bereavement in others with whom they had close interpersonal connections, and the bereavement lasts on an individual basis for as long as those survivors continue to grieve and mourn. Only about one in two bereft individuals (46.7%) reported that the decedent's death was expected (Rosner et al. 2021). This is a bit at odds with the reality that most deaths are due to known natural causes (e.g., cardiovascular disease, cancer) and therefore, perhaps, expected. It also suggests that many bereft individuals may not have been fully aware of decedents' health conditions, or risks associated with decedents' health conditions, near the times of their deaths. Lack of awareness or understanding of the health condition of a significant person near the end of life may adversely affect a bereft individual's adaptation to the loss. This speaks to the potential of clinical attention to family caregivers' mental and emotional preparation for an impending death as a potential way to promote bereavement adjustment. Although only a small minority (11.7%) of bereft individuals utilized health care services because of their grief, nearly two-thirds (63.3%) of those with a probable DSM-5-TR diagnosis of PGD did so (Rosner et al. 2021). This suggests that bereft individuals with PGD often are aware of their bereavement difficulties and actively seek help for coping with their grief.

Prevalence of PGD

A variety of studies have estimated the prevalence of a grief disorder akin to PGD in various populations. However, an overwhelming majority of those studies used methods to assess PGD that are neither consonant nor readily reconcilable with the DSM-5-TR or ICD-11 diagnoses for PGD.

The prevalence of PGD within a given population depends on the criteria for PGD applied, as well as specification of the population in which the criteria are applied. Because PGD is restricted to bereavement, it is natural and common practice to consider the prevalence of PGD within bereaved populations. Ideally, one would estimate the prevalence of PGD within a given population using newly minted DSM or ICD criteria for PGD in a representative sample of that population. However, given that PGD is a new diagnostic entity, and almost all epidemiological research on PGD to date has been conducted using convenience sampling, one should interpret cautiously the literature on the prevalence of PGD.

Prevalence of PGD Using DSM-5-TR and ICD-11 Criteria

Two recent studies have used assessments of PGD concordant with the present DSM-5-TR or ICD-11 diagnostic criteria for PGD and therefore provide the current best estimates of the prevalence of PGD. The Rosner et al. 2021 study designed to estimate prevalence of PGD consistent with DSM-5-TR and ICD-11 criteria in a representative sample of the general German population found a probable 3.3% prevalence of PGD by DSM-5-TR criteria and 4.2% by ICD-11 criteria (which requires just one or more accessory symptoms) among bereaved individuals (n=914; 36.6% of the total sample of 2,498).

A second study (Prigerson et al. 2021), designed to introduce and validate the Prolonged Grief 13 Revised (PG-13-R, a version of the PG-13 grief intensity scale revised to correspond to the DSM-5-TR criteria for PGD), reported the prevalence of PGD by DSM-5-TR criteria in three independent community-based studies of bereft populations in the United States (the Yale Bereavement Study; Prigerson et al. 2009), the Netherlands (the Utrecht Bereavement Study; Boelen et al. 2015), and the United Kingdom (the Oxford Grief Study; Smith and Ehlers 2020). In the Yale Bereavement Study, community-dwelling bereft individuals, primarily widowed, were recruited to participate in a field trial of consensus criteria for PGD. In the Utrecht Bereavement Study, bereft individuals seeking help (not necessarily grief-related) were recruited by mental health care providers to examine the role of cognitive behavioral factors in bereavement adjustment. In the Oxford Grief Study, bereft individuals were recruited via location-targeted social media advertising and the Google content network to participate in an investigation of loss-related memories, appraisals, and coping strategies in relation to the development and maintenance of PGD. The prevalences of PGD using DSM-5-TR criteria in the Yale, Utrecht, and Oxford study samples were 4.4%, 15.3%, and 10.9%, respectively. The prevalence of PGD in the Yale Bereavement Study (4.4%) is comparable to that in the Rosner et al. (2021) study (3.3%). This suggests that the prevalence of PGD, at least in developed Western societies, may be approximately 4% (Figure 6–1). The rates of PGD in the Utrecht Bereavement Study (15.3%) and the Oxford Grief Study (10.9%) suggest that the prevalence of PGD within help-seeking or information-seeking bereft populations is approximately three times greater than that of more general bereft populations.

Prevalence of PGD Using *PLoS Medicine* (or Closely Related) Criteria

Various studies have reported the prevalence of PGD in bereaved populations based on diagnostic assessments using the criteria for PGD originally proposed in *PLoS Medicine* (Prigerson et al. 2009). Because they served as a starting point and foundation for the current DSM-5-TR and ICD-11 formulations of PGD, the *PLoS Medicine* criteria (Prigerson et al. 2009) have extensive overlap and substantial agreement with both DSM-5-TR and

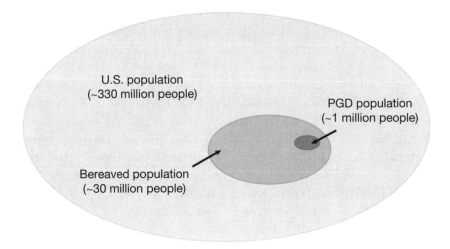

Figure 6–1. Estimated bereaved and PGD subpopulations in the United States circa 2020.

ICD-11 diagnostic assessments for PGD. For example, in the Yale Bereavement Study sample, the prevalence of PGD was 3.3% according to the *PLoS Medicine* criteria (Prigerson et al. 2009) and 4.4% according to the DSM-5-TR criteria (Prigerson et al. 2021). Thus, rates of PGD estimated using the *PLoS Medicine* criteria are likely to be comparable to, and reflective of, those that might have been estimated using the DSM-5-TR or ICD-11 criteria for PGD.

In a nationwide sample of bereft adults in China (*N*=445) (He et al. 2014), 1.8% met criteria for PGD (PG-13, *PLoS Medicine* diagnostic criteria). However, the study sample was not representative of the general Chinese bereft population, and the rate of PGD within the study sample most likely underestimates the prevalence of PGD therein. Participants were recruited from university, hospital, and community settings. Individuals within the study sample, many of whom were university students, were undoubtedly much younger (mean age 27.6 years) and much more likely to be bereft by the loss of a grandparent (58.2%) than the general Chinese bereft population. Given that middle aged adults, compared with young adults, are more likely to be bereft by the loss of a parent, spouse/partner, or child as opposed to a grandparent, and that these losses most likely pose greater risks for PGD than the loss of a grandparent, it is plausible that the prevalence of PGD in the general Chinese bereft population is comparable to that in the general German bereft population (i.e., ~3.3%) (Rosner et al. 2021).

It is common for segments of a general bereft population to have rates of PGD that are substantially higher than that of the general population. For example, in a sample of bereft *shidu* parents—those who had lost their only child and remained childless—in China (*N*=1,030) (Zhou et al. 2020), 20.9% met criteria for PGD (PG-13, *PLoS Medicine* diagnostic criteria) nearly 10 years after the loss, on average. In a sample of female refugees seeking asylum in Germany primarily from Syria, Afghanistan, Eritrea, Iran, Iraq, and Somalia (*N*=85) (Steil et al. 2019), 9.4% met criteria for PGD (PG-13, *PLoS Medicine* diagnostic criteria). Thus, bereft individuals who experience personally consequential losses (e.g., loss of one's only child in a culture in which children are expected to care for parents into their old age) or who are displaced from their countries of origin to escape war or persecution are likely to have higher rates of PGD than the general population.

Studies of bereft individuals who served as family caregivers of patients who died of terminal illnesses suggest that the prevalence of PGD within this subpopulation is comparable to that of more general populations. For example, in a Taiwanese study of bereft caregivers of deceased cancer patients (*N*=493) (Tsai et al. 2016), ~2% met criteria for PGD (PG-13, *PLoS Medicine* diagnostic criteria) 13–24 months after the loss. In an Australian study of family caregivers of cancer patients admitted to palliative care services (*N*=85) (Zordan et al. 2019), 4.7% met criteria for PGD (PG-13, *PLoS Medicine* diagnostic criteria) 37 months after the loss. Thus, overall, family caregivers of patients with terminal illnesses appear to have nearly average risk for developing PGD as a result of the death of those patients.

Several studies have investigated the prevalence of PGD in populations bereft because of genocide or genocidal war. In a study of orphaned (*n*=206) and widowed (*n*=194) survivors who had lost a parent or husband during the 1994 Rwandan genocide (Schaal et al. 2010), 8.0% met criteria for PGD (PG-13, *PLoS Medicine* diagnostic criteria) 12 years later. In a study of survivors who lost a family member during the Khmer Rouge genocide in Cambodia (1975–1979; *N*=775) (Stammel et al. 2013), 14.3% met criteria for PGD (Inventory of Complicated Grief Revised [ICG-R], diagnostic criteria prior to *PLoS Medicine*) (Prigerson et al. 2008) three decades later. In a study of bereaved young Kosovar adults exposed to Kosovo war–related trauma and death of a father in childhood or adolescence (*N*=179) (Morina et al. 2011), 34.6% met criteria for PGD (PG-13, *PLoS Medicine* diagnostic criteria) a decade later. In a related study of mothers widowed by the Kosovo war (*N*=100) (Morina and Emmelkamp 2012), 69.0% met criteria for PGD (PG-13, *PLoS Medicine* diagnostic criteria) a decade later. These studies reveal not only how prevalent PGD is within these subpopulations but also that individuals affected with PGD experience intense grief decades after losses.

Two studies examined the prevalence of PGD among bereft individuals who lost a family member during the 2004 tsunami in Southeast Asia. In a study of bereft survivors in five tsunami-affected coastal villages in India ($N=351$) (Rajkumar et al. 2015), 25.9% met criteria for PGD (diagnostic criteria prior to *PLoS Medicine*) (Prigerson and Maciejewski 2005) 9 months after the tsunami. In a study of bereft Norwegians who had lost a close family member during the tsunami ($N=94$), among 66 who were not directly exposed to the tsunami (Kristensen et al. 2015), 14.9% and 11.7% met criteria for PGD (ICG, diagnostic criteria prior to *PLoS Medicine*) (Prigerson et al. 2008) 2 and 6 years later, respectively. Among 28 Norwegians directly exposed to the tsunami, 21.4% and 17.9% met criteria for PGD 2 and 6 years later, respectively. Thus, bereft native Indian and bereft Norwegian visitor survivors of the 2004 Southeast Asia tsunami had comparable rates of PGD.

Prevalence of PGD Using Latent Class Growth Analysis

Although the DSM-5-TR and ICD-11 criteria are designed to assess PGD at a single point in time, in principle it is possible to identify individuals with PGD by assessing the intensity of their grief over extended periods of time. That is, individuals with long, uninterrupted periods of intense grief meet the conceptual definition of prolonged grief. A longitudinal study of grief associated with bereavement due to sudden parental loss in children 7–18 years old, using a latent class growth analysis, found that 10.4% had elevated, intense grief (modified ICG-R; continuous score measure) (Melhem et al. 2007) over a period of 2 years (Melhem et al. 2011). Thus, the prevalence of PGD among children in this population appears comparable to that of other distressed populations.

Meta-analyses of Prevalence of PGD Using Various Criteria and Bereaved Populations

Meta-analyses examining the prevalence of PGD to date (Djelantik et al. 2020; Lundorff et al. 2017) have used a variety of methods for identifying cases of PGD in a variety of bereaved populations. As a result of this heterogeneity, the bottom-line, aggregate prevalence rates for PGD preclude clear interpretation.

In a meta-analysis of 14 studies of bereavement as a result of nonviolent deaths (Lundorff et al. 2017), the pooled prevalence of PGD was found to be ~ 10%; in a meta-analysis of 25 studies of bereavement as a result of unnatural deaths (e.g., accidents, natural or human-caused disasters, suicide, homicide) (Lundorff et al. 2017), the pooled prevalence of PGD was found to be ~50%. Many studies included in these meta-analyses did not use DSM-5-TR or closely related assessments of PGD; thus, the pooled prevalence of PGD in each of these meta-analyses likely overestimates PGD as now defined in DSM-5-TR. Despite these caveats, it is almost certain that bereft populations exposed to unexpected, unnatural, or violent deaths, as opposed to those exposed to nonviolent deaths, have much higher rates of PGD.

Risk and Protective Factors for Developing PGD

Whereas the prevalence of PGD is sensitive to the diagnostic criteria used and the populations studied, assessments of risk and protective factors for PGD within specific studies (i.e., using common assessments of grief disorder within specified populations) are likely to be more robust. Indeed, because PGD may be characterized as a continued experience of intense grief long after the death of a significant person in one's life, greater severity of grief (as a dimensional construct) many months or years after the loss may reasonably be associated with greater probability of meeting criteria for PGD.

Sociodemographic and Circumstantial Risk Factors and Protective Factors for PGD

Studies in various cultural settings have repeatedly found that the death of a child or spouse (as opposed to parents) is associated with greater risk for developing PGD, and that deaths resulting from foreseeable as opposed to unforeseeable causes, as well as greater age of the decedent, are associated with lower risk for developing PGD (Figure 6–2). For example, in a study of bereaved Chinese adults (He et al. 2014), in a stepwise regression analysis that produced a model of the strongest predictors of severity of grief symptoms, grief symptom severity was significantly associated with loss of a child compared with loss of a parent, loss of a spouse compared with loss of a parent, and traumatic compared with medical cause of death; and it was inversely associated with the age of the decedent. These findings are consistent with those of a longitudinal study of family caregivers of cancer patients admitted to palliative care services in Australia (Thomas et al. 2014), in which severity of grief symptoms in the caregiver months after the death of the patient was significantly associated with the caregiver living with the patient as opposed to elsewhere and the loss of a spouse as opposed to a parent, and

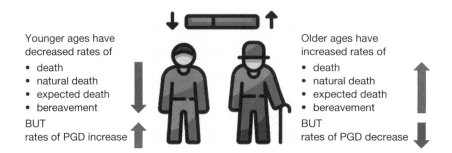

Younger ages have
decreased rates of
- death
- natural death
- expected death
- bereavement

BUT
rates of PGD increase

Older ages have
increased rates of
- death
- natural death
- expected death
- bereavement

BUT
rates of PGD decrease

Figure 6–2.   Relationship of age to risk of bereavement and PGD.

again inversely associated with the age of the decedent. In a population-based Danish survey of family caregivers of patients with terminal illnesses (Nielsen et al. 2017), loss of a partner compared with other losses (primarily of a parent) was associated with greater likelihood of grief disorder. Thus, generally, deaths of children or spouses/partners as opposed to those of other kinship relationships, and unanticipated as opposed to anticipated deaths, elevate risk for developing PGD. (It is important to note that the perception of a loss as being unexpected or unanticipated may be a function of the mourner's difficulty in accepting the dying or death of the loved one.)

A general population study of bereft individuals in Japan (Fujisawa et al. 2010), one consistent with the more general findings that widowed persons and those bereft by unexpected deaths of close others are at greater risk for developing PGD, found that the location of a death and frequency of contact with the decedent near the end of life are also related to the likelihood of developing PGD. In a sample of bereaved community-dwelling individuals ages 40–79 randomly sampled from census tracts in Japan (*N*=969), loss of a spouse (as opposed to a parent), death due to stroke or heart disease (as opposed to cancer), death in hospice or in a care facility (as opposed to at home), and unexpected death were each associated with significantly greater likelihood of grief disorder; death in a general hospital as opposed to at home and no or infrequent contact with the decedent near the end of life were associated with a significantly lower likelihood of grief disorder. It may be the case that individuals who feel very close to decedents desire to care for them at home near the end of their lives. Thus deaths in general hospitals may be indicative of lower degrees of closeness with the bereaved and thus lower risk for developing PGD; deaths in hospice facilities may trouble individuals who feel close to decedents and thus increase risk for developing PGD. Bereft individuals with no or infrequent contact with decedents near the end of their lives are perhaps less likely to have been very close to them in other ways as well, thus placing them at lower risk for developing PGD.

In some cases, risks for developing PGD may be best understood in specific cultural contexts. For example, in the multiple linear regression analysis of severity of grief symptoms of *shidu* parents bereaved by the death of an only child ($N=1,030$) (Zhou et al. 2020), grief symptom severity was significantly associated with being female (a mother) versus being male, residing in a rural versus an urban area, younger age, lower income, and higher number of chronic physical illnesses. In China, children are not only expected but required to care for their aging parents, which lends some insight into these specific risks for developing PGD within this bereft subpopulation: loss of an only child in the present also has the significance of being the loss of their sole primary caregiver in later life. Thus, sociodemographic factors that pose risks for developing PGD among *shidu* individuals appear to be, perhaps not coincidentally, the same sociodemographic factors that might predict hardship for the bereft parent in late life.

In an online survey of racially and ethnically diverse bereaved students ($N=899$) at three colleges at the City University of New York (Goldsmith et al. 2008), Black or Asian (as opposed to white) race, greater degree of anxious and avoidant attachment, and history of anxiety, depression, and trauma were associated with higher rates of PGD; loss of a parent, sibling, or friend (as opposed to a grandparent), degree of closeness to the decedent, violent death (accident, homicide, suicide) as opposed to death from medical illness, and sudden/unexpected death were also associated with higher rates of PGD.

In a study of the effects of exposure to deaths by suicide on mental health (Cerel et al. 2017), more numerous individuals known who died by suicide, greater perceived impact of the most salient death by suicide on one's life, and greater perceived closeness to that decedent were each significantly associated with greater likelihood of PGD. The rate of PGD was only 1.0% in the low-closeness group but 19.9% in the high-closeness group. Thus, repeated exposures to deaths by suicide, perceived disruption in one's life due to a death by suicide, and perceived closeness to a person who has died by suicide increase the likelihood that an individual bereft by suicide will develop PGD.

Modifiable Risk Factors and Protective Factors for PGD

Whereas fixed or stable attributes such as sociodemographic characteristics of the bereft and the decedent and circumstances of the death may be interpreted as risk factors or protective factors for PGD in analysis and interpretation of cross-sectional data, determination of mutable psychological, social, behavioral, and physical health factors as risk or protective factors for PGD requires analysis and interpretation of longitudinal data. Because these attributes may be consequences, and not causes, of PGD, it is important to establish that present states of these factors predict future occurrences of PGD.

Longitudinal studies of family caregivers of patients with terminal illnesses, which allow assessment of caregiver factors before the death of the close other, provide much of what is known about modifiable antecedent predictors of PGD. For example, in a large, prospective, population-based Danish survey of family caregivers of patients with terminal illnesses (N=2,215 bereaved within 6 months who completed a postloss follow-up questionnaire) (Nielsen et al. 2017), greater likelihood of grief disorder at 6 months after the loss was significantly associated with preloss grief and depressive symptoms in the caregiver. In a study of Swedish family members (N=128) of patients with advanced incurable illnesses receiving palliative care in their own homes (Holm et al. 2019), preloss grief was significantly associated with continuing grief 6 months after the death of the patient. Thus, family caregivers who are grief-stricken or depressed while in their caregiving role are at greater risk for developing PGD in bereavement.

In a study in Taiwan that used generalized estimating equation multiple logistic regression analysis of predictors of prolonged grief for bereaved family caregivers over the first 2 years after a terminally ill cancer patient's death (N=493) (Tsai et al. 2016), greater likelihood of PGD was significantly associated with caregiver depressive symptoms preloss and negative perceptions about the circumstances of the death; PGD was significantly inversely associated with subjective caregiver burden and postloss social support. Thus, both negative affect in the caregiving role and negative cognitions about the circumstances of the death were found to be psychological risk factors for developing PGD. Caregivers who found their caregiving role to be more burdensome were less likely to develop PGD (this may be because they felt relieved by, or found it easier to accept, the death of the close other). Caregivers with greater social support after the loss were found to be less likely to develop PGD, strengthening the notion that meaningful social engagement postloss may facilitate more adaptive adjustment to the death of a close other.

In a study in the United States of family members (N=123) of nursing home residents who died with advanced dementia (Givens et al. 2011), family member grief preloss and having lived with the decedent before admission to the nursing home were independently associated with severity of grief 7 months after the death. These risk factors likely reflect the closeness of family members' social-emotional and social-environmental ties to the decedent, making them more likely to be deeply affected by the loss. In a study of spousal caregivers of cancer patients within the United States (N=198) (Miller et al. 2020), poorer mental and physical health and lower degree of active coping in a caregiver before the death of a spouse were significantly associated with greater severity of grief symptoms 6–15 months after the death. Bereft spouses (widowed persons) with preexisting and ongoing mental, physical, and behavioral health challenges have lost their closest allies in their daily struggles.

In an Australian study of family caregivers of cancer patients admitted to palliative care services (N=143 followed 13 months after the loss) (Thomas et al. 2014), higher grief preloss, lower optimism, impact of caregiving on schedule, and poorer family functioning were significantly associated with severity of caregiver grief symptoms 13 months after the loss. These findings highlight that there may well be distinct affective, cognitive, behavioral, and social risk factors for developing PGD.

PGD as a Risk for Subsequent Psychopathology

PGD not only is distressing and disabling but also poses a risk for other forms of psychopathology. In one study (Prigerson et al. 2021) that analyzed three independent bereaved groups from prospective studies of PGD conducted within the United States, the United Kingdom, and the Netherlands, meeting DSM-5-TR criteria for PGD was predictive of subsequent mental disorder (major depressive disorder, generalized anxiety disorder, or PTSD); severity of symptoms of depression and PTSD; suicidality; poorer vitality-, role emotional–, and mental health–related quality of life; and severity of work and social adjustment difficulties. In another study conducted in the Netherlands (Djelantik et al. 2018), in a cross-lagged analysis, severity of PGD symptoms was predictive of severity of PTSD symptoms 1 year later, whereas there was no evidence that severity of PTSD symptoms predicted severity of PGD symptoms. These studies suggest that PGD may be a gateway to broader psychopathology in bereavement, and thus that identification and treatment of PGD may prevent an array of mental health and mental health–related problems.

References

American Psychiatric Association: Diagnostic and Statistical Manual of Mental Disorders, 5th Edition, Text Revision. Washington, DC, American Psychiatric Association, 2022

Boelen PA, de Keijser J, Smid G: Cognitive-behavioral variables mediate the impact of violent loss on post-loss psychopathology. Psychol Trauma 7(4):382–390, 2015 26147521

Cerel J, Maple M, van de Venne J, et al: Suicide exposure in the population: perceptions of impact and closeness. Suicide Life Threat Behav 47(6):696–708, 2017 28150414

Djelantik AAAMJ, Smid GE, Kleber RJ, Boelen PA: Do prolonged grief disorder symptoms predict post-traumatic stress disorder symptoms following bereavement? A cross-lagged analysis. Compr Psychiatry 80:65–71, 2018 29055233

Djelantik AAAMJ, Smid GE, Mroz A, et al: The prevalence of prolonged grief disorder in bereaved individuals following unnatural losses: systematic review and meta regression analysis. J Affect Disord 265:146–156, 2020 32090736

Fujisawa D, Miyashita M, Nakajima S, et al: Prevalence and determinants of complicated grief in general population. J Affect Disord 127(1–3):352–35, 2010 20580096

Givens JL, Prigerson HG, Kiely DK, et al: Grief among family members of nursing home residents with advanced dementia. Am J Geriatr Psychiatry 19(6):543–550, 2011 21606897

Goldsmith B, Morrison RS, Vanderwerker LC, Prigerson HG: Elevated rates of prolonged grief disorder in African Americans. Death Stud 32(4):352–365, 2008 18850684

He L, Tang S, Yu W, et al: The prevalence, comorbidity and risks of prolonged grief disorder among bereaved Chinese adults. Psychiatry Res 219(2):347–352, 2014 24924526

Holm M, Årestedt K, Alvariza A: Associations between predeath and postdeath grief in family caregivers in palliative home care. J Palliat Med 22(12):1530–1535, 2019 31225778

Kristensen P, Weisaeth L, Hussain A, Heir T: Prevalence of psychiatric disorders and functional impairment after loss of a family member: a longitudinal study after the 2004 Tsunami. Depress Anxiety 32(1):49–56, 2015

Lundorff M, Holmgren H, Zachariae R, et al: Prevalence of prolonged grief disorder in adult bereavement: a systematic review and meta-analysis. J Affect Disord 212:138–149, 2017 28167398

Melhem NM, Moritz G, Walker M, et al: Phenomenology and correlates of complicated grief in children and adolescents. J Am Acad Child Adolesc Psychiatry 46(4):493–499, 2007 17420684

Melhem NM, Porta G, Shamseddeen W, et al: Grief in children and adolescents bereaved by sudden parental death. Arch Gen Psychiatry 68(9):911–919, 2011 21893658; erratum in JAMA Psychiatry 76:1319, 2019 21893658

Miller LM, Utz RL, Supiano K, et al: Health profiles of spouse caregivers: the role of active coping and the risk for developing prolonged grief symptoms. Soc Sci Med 266:113455, 2020 33126099

Morina N, Emmelkamp PM: Mental health outcomes of widowed and married mothers after war. Br J Psychiatry 200(2):158–159, 2012 22116978

Morina N, von Lersner U, Prigerson HG: War and bereavement: consequences for mental and physical distress. PLoS One 6(7):e22140, 2011 21765944

Nielsen MK, Neergaard MA, Jensen AB, et al: Predictors of complicated grief and depression in bereaved caregivers: a nationwide prospective cohort study. J Pain Symptom Manage 53(3):540–550, 2017 28042073

Prigerson HG, Maciejewski PK: A call for sound empirical testing and evaluation of criteria for complicated grief proposed for DSM-V. Omega 52(1):9–19, 2005

Prigerson HG, Vanderwerker LC, Maciejewski PK: A case for inclusion of prolonged grief disorder in DSM-V, in Handbook of Bereavement Research and Practice. Edited by Stroebe MS, Hansson R, Schut H, Stroebe W. Washington, DC, American Psychological Association, 2008, pp 165–186

Prigerson HG, Horowitz MJ, Jacobs SC, et al: Prolonged grief disorder: psychometric validation of criteria proposed for DSM-V and ICD-11. PLoS Med 6(8):e1000121, 2009 19652695

Prigerson HG, Boelen PA, Xu J, et al: Validation of the new DSM-5-TR criteria for prolonged grief disorder and the PG-13-Revised (PG-13-R) scale. World Psychiatry 20(1):96–106, 2021 33432758

Rajkumar AP, Mohan TS, Tharyan P: Lessons from the 2004 Asian tsunami: nature, prevalence and determinants of prolonged grief disorder among tsunami survivors in South Indian coastal villages. Int J Soc Psychiatry 61(7):645–652, 2015 25687577

Rosner R, Comtesse H, Vogel A, Doering BK: Prevalence of prolonged grief disorder. J Affect Disord 287:301–307, 2021 33812243

Schaal S, Jacob N, Dusingizemungu JP, Elbert T: Rates and risks for prolonged grief disorder in a sample of orphaned and widowed genocide survivors. BMC Psychiatry 10:55, 2010 20604936

Smith KV, Ehlers A: Cognitive predictors of grief trajectories in the first months of loss: a latent growth mixture model. J Consult Clin Psychol 88(2):93–105, 2020 31556649

Stammel N, Heeke C, Bockers E, et al: Prolonged grief disorder three decades post loss in survivors of the Khmer Rouge regime in Cambodia. J Affect Disord 144(1–2):87–93, 2013 22871529

Steil R, Gutermann J, Harrison O, et al: Prevalence of prolonged grief disorder in a sample of female refugees. BMC Psychiatry 19(1):148, 2019 31088419

Thomas K, Hudson P, Trauer T, et al: Risk factors for developing prolonged grief during bereavement in family carers of cancer patients in palliative care: a longitudinal study. J Pain Symptom Manage 47(3):531–54, 2014 23969327

Tsai W-I, Prigerson HG, Li C-Y, et al: Longitudinal changes and predictors of prolonged grief for bereaved family caregivers over the first 2 years after the terminally ill cancer patient's death. Palliat Med 30(5):495–503, 2016 26311571

Verdery AM, Smith-Greenaway E, Margolis R, Daw J: Tracking the reach of COVID-19 kin loss with a bereavement multiplier applied to the United States. Proc Natl Acad Sci USA 117(30):17695–17701, 2020 32651279

Woolf SH, Chapman DA, Lee JH: COVID-19 as the leading cause of death in the United States. JAMA 325(2):123–124, 2021

World Health Organization: International Statistical Classification of Diseases and Related Health Problems, 11th Revision. Geneva, World Health Organization, 2022

Zhou N, Wen J, Stelzer EM, et al: Prevalence and associated factors of prolonged grief disorder in Chinese parents bereaved by losing their only child. Psychiatry Res 284:112766, 2020 31951871

Zordan RD, Bell ML, Price M, et al: Long-term prevalence and predictors of prolonged grief disorder amongst bereaved cancer caregivers: a cohort study. Palliat Support Care 17(5):507–514, 2019 30767818

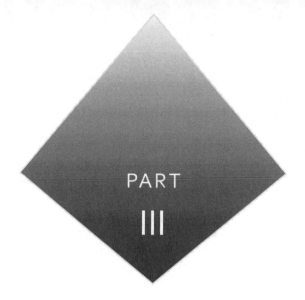

PART

III

Treatment of Prolonged Grief Disorder

7

Treatment of Prolonged Grief Disorder

Natalia Skritskaya, Ph.D.
Meredith Charney, Ph.D.
Naomi M. Simon, M.D.
M. Katherine Shear, M.D.

*I think about the person [who died] so much that it's
    hard to do the things I normally do.*
Memories of the person who died upset me.
I feel I cannot accept the death…
I find myself longing for the person who died.
I can't help feeling angry about [their] death.
I feel that life is empty without [them].
*I feel that it is unfair that I should live when this
    person died.*
I feel bitter over this person's death.
                                  —Inventory of Complicated Grief
                                     (Prigerson et al. 1995, p. 79)

PGD is an important new diagnosis that is estimated to affect millions of people in the United States alone. The life of a person with
prolonged grief disorder (PGD) is filled with thoughts and feelings—such as
those in this chapter's epigraph—that match items on the Inventory of Com-

plicated Grief (Prigerson et al. 1995). The condition is associated with considerable distress and impairment, including elevated rates of suicidality (Boelen and Prigerson 2007; Latham and Prigerson 2004). Caught in a seemingly endless loop of suffering, without effective treatment, PGD can persist for decades, robbing sufferers of their own lives and isolating them from friends and loved ones. Untreated, it can bring a person's life to a standstill.

Fortunately there is now a solid body of research, much of it reviewed in this handbook, to guide clinicians. *Complicated grief therapy* (CGT) was the first targeted treatment shown to be efficacious (Shear et al. 2005). This chapter describes CGT, now named *prolonged grief disorder therapy* (PGDT) (Mauro et al. 2022), including an overview of the approach and a description of the course of treatment illustrated with a client case history. Additionally, we provide a summary of other therapeutic approaches, including several that have the support of randomized controlled trials (RCTs) and some promising pilot and case studies. We also discuss a possible role for medication in PGD treatment, although evidence-based psychotherapies are the first-line treatment, as to date there is not yet available a pharmacotherapy with RCT-level evidence specifically for PGD (e.g., Shear, Reynolds, Simon, Zisook 2016).

As described earlier in this handbook, the syndrome now called prolonged grief disorder has had different names. Examples include *unresolved grief, traumatic grief, complicated grief,* and *persistent complex bereavement disorder* (e.g., American Psychiatric Association 2013; DeVaul and Zisook 1976; Horowitz et al. 1993; Prigerson et al. 2009). None of them exactly matches the criteria used in DSM-5-TR (American Psychiatric Association 2022) or previously proposed criteria with the term *prolonged grief disorder* (Prigerson et al. 2009). However, each criteria set identifies individuals who would likely meet the published DSM-5-TR criteria for PGD, and all were included in research for the new diagnosis. In our own work, we have referred to the condition using different names. Following Prigerson et al. (1997) at the time we developed the treatment, we used the name *traumatic grief therapy* (TGT; Shear et al. 2001), and then, also following Prigerson's work, we began using *complicated grief therapy* (Shear et al. 2005). To minimize ongoing confusion around different names, we refer to the treatment as *prolonged grief disorder therapy* (PGDT) in the current chapter and moving forward.[1]

---

[1] In a reanalysis of our study data (Shear, Reynolds, Simon, Zisook 2016) using (proposed) DSM-5 PGD criteria, most of the original study sample met criteria for DSM-5-TR PGD, and treatment outcomes did not differ from original findings (Mauro et al. 2022).

PGDT: An Overview

PGDT is an integrative short-term psychotherapy for PGD, a loss-related stress-response syndrome with characteristics partly resembling posttraumatic stress disorder (PTSD) (Stroebe et al. 2001). We developed this approach by modifying elements of Foa's well-validated *prolonged exposure* for PTSD (Shear 2006), including daily symptom monitoring (grief monitoring), imaginal exposure (revisiting of the story of the death through imagination and projected dialog), and in vivo exposure (situational revisiting of reminders of the loss). We developed one rating scale for grief-related avoidance (Shear et al. 2007) and another rating scale for possible PGD-related cognitions (Skritskaya et al. 2017). Considering that the grief syndrome we were treating occurred in response to the death of someone close, we turned to attachment theory to understand its roots. It appeared that pathognomonic grief symptoms could be understood as manifestations of attachment/caregiving system activation that occurs in response to separation from a deceased close attachment. Additionally, in his seminal book on loss, Bowlby (1980) posited that the stress of such a loss typically engendered a protective response comprising common defensive coping strategies. These coping responses are often helpful in the short run but may become problematic when overly prominent and persistent. As Bowlby observed,

> The criteria that most clearly distinguish healthy forms of defensive process from pathological ones are the length of time during which they persist and the extent to which they influence a part only of mental functioning or come to dominate it completely. (Bowlby 1980, p. 140)

The persistence of overly influential defensive responses characterizes patients with PGD.

Bowlby (1980) further described the process of successfully mourning a loss as requiring acceptance of its finality, revision of the attachment working model, and redefinition of life goals and plans. Because the term *mourning* now generally refers to the outward expression of grief, we describe this process as *adapting to* the loss. Adapting, so defined, is fundamentally a learning process that, when accomplished, reduces the frequency, intensity, and duration of grief symptoms and fosters comprehension and integration of the finality and consequences of the loss into ongoing psychological functioning.

While unique to each person and each loss, the process of adapting generally entails accepting the reality of the loss and restoring the capacity for well-being. Adaptation can be impeded or derailed by overly influential defensive processes, as alluded to by Bowlby (1980). When adapting is derailed, grief remains strong and pervasive. Based on this conceptualization, we designed PGDT to focus on fostering adaptation and addressing the derailers. To accomplish this, we operationalized the process of adapting as seven core steps and organized the treatment to address them, with seven core procedures and treatment themes. We manualized the treatment as a 16-session semistructured integrative intervention that has a planned sequence and a series of specific procedures.

A PGDT therapist introduces procedures that begin the process of rebuilding capacity for well-being and then the procedures that target the more emotionally challenging acceptance of the reality. In three RCTs sponsored by the National Institute of Mental Health, the treatment has been compared to proven efficacious treatments for depression. We specifically considered depression-focused treatments because we found depression to be the most common misdiagnosis among the patients we treated. Results of these studies were consistent, showing clinically and statistically significant superiority of PGDT over either interpersonal therapy for depression (Shear et al. 2005, 2014) or antidepressant medication, citalopram (Shear, Reynolds, Simon, Zisook 2016). More details of these studies and their results are described after a case-based presentation of the 16-session therapy.

Introducing the 16-Session Therapy: A Case-Based Approach

PGDT is delivered in four phases: Getting Started (sessions 1–3), Core Revisiting Sequence (sessions 4–9), Midcourse Review (Session 10), and Closing Sequence (sessions 11–16). In the section that follows, we introduce Casey, a bereaved mother grieving her son, and then walk through the four phases of her treatment and its core procedures and themes, explaining what we do, how we do it, and some of the challenges a therapist faces in working with patients such as Casey. Of note, we have used PGDT successfully following the death of any close friend or family member for a variety of causes, including terminal illness or violence. The circumstances of the death do not appear to moderate treatment effects (Na et al. 2021).

Case Example: Casey

Casey is a 57-year-old woman with a lovely smile and deep sadness in her eyes. She appears composed entering the therapist's office but is quick to get teary while explaining what brought her in. She does not understand what is happening, why her grief does not get better. It has been more than 4 years since her son Daniel died of accidental overdose, but she can still barely function. She manages to go to work, but otherwise does not want to see anyone or leave her house. She feels lost and doesn't know how much longer she can go on like this. Casey tells the therapist that, honestly, she doesn't believe anyone can help her, but she doesn't know what else to do and is willing to give this therapy a try.

Getting Started (Sessions 1–3)

The first three sessions focus on building the foundation of treatment by gathering information about the client's experience of loss and grief and establishing a therapeutic alliance. The sessions introduce procedures for working with Theme 1, understanding grief; Theme 2, managing strong emotions; Theme 3, seeing a promising future; and Theme 4, strengthening relationships.

Session 1

PGDT Session 1 focuses on reviewing the patient's history, including childhood experiences and adult life before the death in question. The therapist is interested in the patient's important relationships and their personal and social strengths and vulnerabilities. The therapist also reviews the patient's relationship with the deceased, the story of the death, and the patient's experiences since the loss. At the end of Session 1, interval activities are introduced, beginning with grief monitoring.

Casey's History

Casey was one of six children. Money was scarce in this large family; her parents were busy and did not have much time for affection. As one of the oldest, she was expected to help raise her siblings and take care of the house. She was taught to do her best at whatever she started. She was a good student and enjoyed school. She did well, completed college, and got an accounting job at a big company. A couple of years later, she married Tomas, and Daniel was born. She continued to work because she and Tomas needed the money and also because she felt she was good at what she did. Her relationship with Tomas faltered, but she loved Daniel and stayed with Tomas because of their son. She divided her energy between Daniel and her work. She and her son were close, and they were a lot alike: they got each other's jokes and shared creative passions. She said he was her "mini-me." When he started high school, Daniel started experimenting with drugs, and their life became a roller coaster of rehab stays and periods of sobriety and relapse. Casey and Tomas struggled to get Daniel back on track. However, their marriage was not strong; they saw his problem very differently and the relationship did not survive. Sadly, she lost Daniel as well when he was only 25. On a winter night almost 4 years before, a police officer called and asked her to come to the station, where they informed her of Daniel's death by overdose. She was devastated and continues to feel lost and unable to find her way forward.

Casey's PGD Symptoms

More than 4 years after Daniel's death, his things are still packed in boxes in Casey's attic; she cannot bring herself to go through them. She avoids all social occasions, including seeing her friends, because it takes too much energy to put on a "happy face." She also avoids places and situations that remind her of Daniel because it feels like too much to bear: the cemetery, the part of town where he worked, restaurants they liked, even music and photography they both enjoyed. Her home feels sad and empty, but it seems safer than anyplace else, so she mostly stays home. She continues to go to work but does only the bare minimum to get by. She is disappointed in herself for not being able to cope with this loss after so much time. She thinks she should be improving by now, that she should stop grieving all the time. She does not recognize herself anymore. Who is this weak person? Casey keeps thinking how she failed as a mother. She should have checked on Daniel more. She keeps thinking that she could have prevented the overdose, that she should have shown him more love and affection when he was younger, and that she should have tried harder in her marriage with Tomas. Sometimes she is angry at the police for not doing more to catch drug dealers and at society at large for not doing more to stop the opioid epidemic. She often thinks she should have died instead of Daniel.

Casey's only respite is in the past; she spends hours daydreaming of happy times they shared when Daniel was younger—traveling, trading jokes, listening to music, and singing. These reveries bring positive feelings, but when they end, the bleak reality hits her anew, almost like Daniel just died. Casey wishes that one day she would just not wake up, so this torture would end. Her strong religious beliefs are all that keep her from trying to take her own life.

Casey begins *grief monitoring* at the end of Session 1. Her therapist explains that monitoring could help her better understand her experience of grief and its triggers in her daily life. The therapist asks Casey to take a few minutes at the end of each day to identify the highest level of grief for that day, rate how high it was on a scale of 1–10, and recall the situation in which it occurred. She repeats the process for the lowest level that day. Then she thinks back over the day overall and records it as a low (1–3), medium (4–6), or high (7–10) grief day. She is asked to bring the grief log to the next session and discuss it with the therapist.

This procedure helps a patient see the way grief waxes and wanes, which is important, especially early in therapy when patients typically imagine that their grief is constantly high. Over time, grief monitoring helps to identify cues that activate grief and specific grief-related emotions. Grief monitoring can also help identify and address derailers and help patients learn effective ways of managing grief when it is activated. Monitoring provides a way of tracking changes in overall grief levels as treatment progresses.

Introducing Casey to the Grief Monitoring Diary

When the therapist introduces the grief monitoring diary, Casey's first comment is that she hates diaries. The therapist explains that this is a different kind of diary; it is about noticing the highs and lows of her daily grief. She does not need to write a lot, if she does not want to. She can just put down a number for her highest moment of grief each day and a number for her lowest moment, along with a brief note about what was happening in those moments. Then, she can put a number for her overall level of grief for that day. Casey is hesitant about this, but since she came to the treatment determined to do her best, whether she liked an assignment or not, she agrees to try it.

At the end of Session 1, the therapist also introduces the idea of building support and encourages the patient to invite someone to Session 3 for a joint session, the purpose of which is to begin to strengthen this relationship and get another perspective on the patient's grief.

Session 2

Reviewing Casey's Grief Monitoring Diary

At the beginning of Session 2, the therapist asks Casey about the diary. "I completed the form," she says as she takes out the page. "I'm not sure if this is how you wanted it." The therapist quickly glances over the form and praises Casey for completing the diary every day. "This is great, you did it just as I've asked you to. I'm impressed! Even though you had your doubts about this assignment, you completed the diary every day! How did it go?" Casey says it wasn't as bad as she expected. The therapist says, "Let's take a look. Your highest grief level for the week was a 9 on Wednesday, with a note 'picture on my phone.' Can you say a little more about that?" Casey says one of the last pictures of her son popped up on her phone unexpectedly, one of those automatic reminders of photos from years ago. She had put all the photos of him away and deleted them from her phone and must have missed this one. Seeing it was like a floodgate opened, memories and pain rushing in, uncontrollably. Her day was ruined; she could not stop thinking about how Daniel did not have to die in this way, and she was flooded with guilt and anger. She went through the rest of the day struggling to keep those emotions under wraps and unable to concentrate on anything else. She was also angry with herself for letting the feelings spiral out of control and anxious about how she could live her life feeling so emotional and vulnerable. She felt like she just wanted to crawl into bed and wait for the day to be over. It was horrible.

The therapist responds, saying that this sounds pretty overwhelming and painful. There were many troubling thoughts and feelings. The therapist thinks it is going to be important to work with these kinds of painful responses to reminders of Daniel. For now, the therapist asks Casey if they could talk a little about the idea that she is angry with herself for letting these feelings spiral out of control. This enables the therapist to introduce some psychoeducation about grief and to say this will be a topic of more discussion later in the session.

The therapist then asks about Casey's lowest grief level that week, and if it is OK to discuss it. Casey responds, "Sure." The therapist says, "Your lowest level for the week was a 4, and that happened on several days. On Thursday it was a 4 and you wrote, "Distracted at work." Casey replies, "It has been quite busy because we are trying to finish up a project. It's a project that I am pretty interested in...." She pauses. "And that's a little surprising." The therapist says, "That's a great observation. It doesn't really surprise me, because people who are experiencing prolonged grief can still experience positive emotions, but I also know that it can be uncomfortable to do so. Sometimes people 'forget' that they were interested." The therapist adds that recognizing this is an important step in starting to restore the capacity for well-being, something else they are going to talk more about in this session. Then the therapist notes that her overall grief ranged from 8 to 9 every day this week and praises Casey again for trying this new tool, asking if she is willing to continue the diary for another week. Casey says she is starting to see how this might be a good thing to do and agrees to keep going.

Psychoeducation.   In Session 2, the therapist spends most of the time discussing the framework for the therapy, which includes a way of understanding grief and adapting to loss. The therapist conveys the view of grief as a natural adaptive response to a meaningful loss, a complex response that encompasses a range of reactions, including temporary changes in psychological and physiological functioning. Knowledge about the attachment, caregiving, and exploration systems provides a context for understanding the bereaved client's specific manifestations of grief. Information gathered during the assessment phase can be very useful here to illustrate these abstract concepts and connect them to a client's reported experiences. The therapist also describes the typical evolution of grief, where it is gradually transformed from an acute form to an integrated form. This occurs as the bereaved person navigates their way through daily experiences to come to terms with the unwanted reality of the loss and its many consequences and to restore a sense of purpose and satisfaction in life, as well as meaningful connections with others. The rationale for attending to restoration of well-being, in addition to facing the loss, is discussed as part of promoting the natural oscillation of grief informed by the dual-process model.

Introducing Aspirational Goals. The third theme—seeing a promising future—is introduced in the last third of Session 2. The therapist introduces procedures for developing an *aspirational goal* as well as engaging in simple rewarding activities. The aspirational goals procedure is a modification of personal goals work used in motivational interviewing. The idea is to help the patient access core values and interests and use them to identify an activity or project that directly connects with an intrinsic interest or value.

Introducing Casey to Aspirational Goals

At the end of the second session, the therapist asks, "If I could wave a magic wand and your grief would be at a manageable level, what would you want for yourself?" "What does it matter? My son is dead!" responds Casey. The therapist agrees that it's difficult to imagine wanting anything after a loss like that. But even though it might not feel like it, her life matters too. One of the goals of this work is to restore the possibility of experiencing well-being and happiness again. The therapist says, "I think you might find this exercise interesting, if you can allow yourself to imagine that you have found a way to come to terms with what happened and your grief is no longer overwhelming your life. Are you willing to try again?" Casey agrees, and the therapist again invites her to consider what she might want for herself. This time Casey pauses and thinks for a few minutes. Then she shakes her head and says, "I don't know. Nothing feels interesting to me.... I can't imagine myself ever feeling less grief." The therapist is quiet as Casey sits, silent and pensive. After a while she continues, "I guess maybe I could take some adult education classes. There are a lot of classes offered online these days; maybe something will catch my interest." She pauses, thinking. "I used to really like photography. I kind of had some natural talent. People told me I was good at it. I remember that I did want to get more training in photography but never had time. Of course, Daniel was into photography, so I'm not sure how I would feel about taking a photography class." The therapist agrees that it might be hard to do something that reminds her of Daniel, but says it might also have an appealing side. The therapist encourages Casey to keep thinking about the idea of taking classes in photography and other potential interests she might pursue.

In Session 2, the therapist also introduces the idea of building into daily life some simple activities that generate positive emotions: things that might be relaxing, fun, interesting, satisfying, or just pleasurable. The therapist asks the patient what things like this she might do. They discuss ideas briefly, and the therapist asks the patient to make a list. In Session 4, they will discuss the list and work on developing a ritual—as short as 5 minutes or as long as she wishes—of doing something from the list every day.

Session 3

Session 3 is usually held with a visitor. Its purpose is to reopen communication between the patient and a close friend or family member, foster understanding, and rebuild a sense of connection between them. Not infrequently, people with PGD feel estranged from others even though those around them want to help. Unfortunately, friends and family members can start to feel helpless and frustrated. This session gives the visitor the opportunity to express affection for the patient, to air some of the frustration they have been feeling, and to learn about PGD and PGDT. If possible, they explore ways to share in supporting the treatment. The therapist learns about the visitor's relationship with the patient before the death and what it has been like since. Patients are often surprised to see how much the visitor still cares; they may also be surprised about aspects of the visitor's perspective on the circumstances of the loss or their level of concern for the patient and their suffering. The visitor is usually very grateful to be included in the session, meet the therapist, and learn a different way of thinking about the grief their friend or family member is experiencing.

Casey Brings Her Friend to Session 3

Casey is hesitant to bring someone to the session. She does not want to inconvenience her friends and also does not feel fully comfortable showing how vulnerable she is. However, after some discussion, she decides to ask her best friend, Jessica, whom she's known most of her life. To Casey's surprise, Jessica needs no convincing to come and is actually pleased to be invited and to hear that Casey is trying grief therapy. Jessica explains that she has been worried about her friend and has been feeling sad that it seems like they've drifted apart since Daniel's death. Jessica says she had practically given up, as Casey has been declining all her invitations to social events and even lunch. Casey had been her closest friend since childhood, but since Daniel died she has not been the same. The witty and adventuresome woman who was often the life of the party is gone, and Jessica is grieving her friend along with her "nephew" Daniel. Casey is shocked to hear this. She tears up as she listens, saying she did not realize she had caused so much pain to her friend. She had started to feel that no one cared anymore—even Jessica— because she felt so alone and did not know how to cope with Daniel's death.

The therapist reflects on Casey's experiences in light of the grief framework used in the treatment. The therapist also answers Jessica's questions about prolonged grief and reviews the main components of the treatment. The therapist asks Casey if she thinks Jessica might be helpful to her as she moves through the treatment. Casey isn't sure, and Jessica asks if they could get together for lunch soon. Both seem excited about the newfound opportunity to reconnect.

Core Revisiting Sequence (Sessions 4–9)

Sessions 4–9 are core revisiting sessions that contain the heart of the loss focus of PGDT. The sessions introduce procedures for working with Theme 5, narrating a coherent story of the death; Theme 6, learning to live with reminders; and Theme 7, connecting with memories. The main procedure for Theme 5 is imaginal revisiting, introduced in Session 4.

Imaginal Revisiting

Imaginal revisiting is a four-step exercise designed to help the patient confront and acknowledge the reality of the death. In Step 1, the patient is asked to close her eyes and visualize the moment she first learned of the death. She tells the story of what happened from that point forward, speaking out loud to the therapist for about 10 minutes. Audio of the patient's story is recorded so that she can listen to it during the week at home. The therapist checks distress levels at regular 2-minute intervals as the patient tells the story, and also whenever it appears that emotionality increases. At the end of the 10 minutes, the therapist asks the patient to open her eyes and report her distress level.

Step 2 entails reflecting on what it was like to tell the story and what she noticed while doing so. The therapist spends the next 10 minutes talking with the patient about these reflections. The therapist listens actively and intervenes if there are opportunities to foster adaptation or address impediments to progress. Step 3 entails setting the story aside. After talking about the revisiting story for 10 minutes, the therapist checks the patient's distress level and asks if she is ready to set the story aside. Patients usually feel ready to do so, but if not, the therapist may do a grounding exercise, for example, inviting the patient to imagine that the story is on a video recording. The therapist asks the patient to imagine that she has just listened to the recording and is now ready to put it away. She visualizes herself doing this as she describes what she's doing out loud. After she imagines playing the video, she imagines taking it out of the device, putting it in a container, and storing it in a place she can access easily (e.g., a dresser drawer). Then they move to Step 4 of the revisiting exercise, the last step, which is planning a rewarding activity to do when she gets home.

These sessions end with a summary, feedback from the patient, and a discussion of plans for the upcoming week. These include daily listening to a recording of the revisiting exercise. The therapist makes plans to talk by phone after the first time the patient listens to the recording.

The imaginal revisiting exercise is repeated during the next three to five sessions. A new audio recording is made each time, and the patient is asked to listen to it during the week. With repetition, the narrative usually becomes more detailed, and distress levels decrease. Patients usually report that after telling or listening to this story a few times, they start to believe that their loved ones are "really gone." Before, they knew it was true but somehow could not really believe it. A feeling of being lighter and more connected to the present is also common.

Casey's Imaginal Revisiting Exercise

Although hesitant at first, Casey follows the therapist's guidance, tells the story of the death in session, and diligently listens to the recording at home every day. It is intense for her, but also a relief in some ways. In repeatedly telling the story in session and then listening to the recording at home, she finds that the events around her son's death become less emotionally potent. She realizes that she can handle the pain and is not afraid to lose control anymore. While she doesn't really like the exercise (as she confided later), it helps to make what happened feel more real and to realize it was not a bad dream.

Telling and listening to this story, Casey becomes freer to think about Daniel's death and events leading up to it. She is reminded how unexpected this death was to everyone, including her son's mental health professionals. She begins to realize that she could not have prevented her son's death. She remembers how difficult it was for her when he was using: the ruined family events, the stolen money, and the loss of the ability to trust him. She also remembers the many ways she tried to help her son during the years he struggled with addiction, and how tirelessly she advocated for his care. Finally, she also recalls that he often expressed his appreciation and told her that she was a good mother. Remembering these things eases her guilt, and she finally understands that she was not responsible for Daniel's death.

Situational Revisiting

Situational revisiting is a procedure to help patients learn to live with reminders of their loss. It targets situations the patient is avoiding by using a procedure similar to in vivo exposure for other disorders in which avoidance is prominent (e.g., panic with agoraphobia, social anxiety disorder, PTSD). The procedure is introduced in Session 5. The patient is asked to begin to make a list of situations—people, places, or things—that she is avoiding because they trigger painful reminders of the loss. In Session 6, the patient discusses the list with the therapist and decides on an activity that entails confronting a situation that the patient can commit to doing every day or as often as possible during the upcoming week. The patient records her grief levels before, during, and after the activity. Usually, distress levels come down during the course of the week, and the patient's comfort level with the situation increases quite noticeably. The therapist then suggests she move to another situation, higher on the distress hierarchy. The process of planning and doing an activity that entails confrontation with this situation is repeated. Usually, this process continues until the end of the treatment, and often the patient leaves therapy with some remaining areas of avoidance that she plans to address over time.

Casey's Situational Avoidance

The therapist reflects on Casey's attempts to control her emotions by avoiding reminders of Daniel's death and asks if it is working well. Casey admits that she does not feel she is successful at not getting triggered. The therapist asks if she would be willing to try a different approach to managing such reminders. Instead of trying to control her grief by avoiding triggers, they would work to help Casey gradually face the reminders and situations she has been avoiding. They first discuss some situations she has been avoiding and make a list of them in order of difficulty. The list includes listening to her favorite music, looking at pictures of her son, and going out to eat, especially in their favorite restaurant. Casey feels that listening to a song that she likes and that reminds her of Daniel would be challenging but doable. She agrees to listen to it every day, and at the next session tells the therapist that it did get easier with repetition.

One of the most difficult situations on the list is going back to their favorite restaurant, which Casey rated as 95 out of 100. With the therapist, she discusses ways to adjust the situation to make it more approachable. First, for a week Casey just drives by the restaurant. When that becomes easier, she parks near the restaurant and sits in her car for a few minutes. Eventually, she is able to get out of her car and walk to the restaurant to look at the menu in the window. Finally, she and her friend Jessica have lunch there one day. When Casey comes to her next session, she is brimming with excitement. She explains that she and Jessica had a great time at the restaurant; she had forgotten how amazing the food was and how much she liked the staff. During the remainder of the treatment, with increased confidence and success, she begins to address other situations on her hierarchy.

Work With Memories and Pictures

Work with memories and pictures begins in Session 6. The therapist asks the patient to complete the first of a set of five memories questionnaires. The first questionnaire focuses on positive memories such as the deceased person's most likeable characteristics, the most enjoyable times with the person, what this person added to the patient's life, and things the patient loved most about the person. The patient continues to write about positive memories after sessions 6, 7, and 8, and then after Session 9, she is invited to think about the "not-so-positive" things about the person and their relationship. After Session 10, she completes a questionnaire about both positive and not-so-positive memories of the person who died. The patient brings the completed memories form to the next session, along with pictures if she wishes. The therapist spends a few minutes in the session reading and talking about the memories and looking at the pictures. The last theme, connecting with memories, begins in this way, and continues into the closing sequence with the final exercise, an imaginal conversation with the person who died. This is generally done in Session 11.

Midcourse Review and Closing Sequence (Sessions 10–16)

Session 10 is devoted to a review of the treatment to date and planning for the remaining sessions. The therapist reviews the PGDT model, discusses it with the patient, and considers what has changed and what still needs work. They discuss progress with situational revisiting, rebuilding support, and aspirational goals. The therapist and patient work collaboratively to plan the last phase of treatment.

The last six sessions of PGDT are used to complete and consolidate treatment gains and discuss thoughts and feelings about treatment termination. The loss-oriented component focuses on helping the patient make peace with the finality of the loss and the permanence of grief, understand what the loss means to them, and feel a sense of connection with the deceased. The restoration-oriented component focuses on helping the patient continue to plan or begin to implement an aspirational goal, build rewarding activities into daily life, and continue to foster a sense of relatedness to other people. Usually by this point in treatment, there is a shift toward restoration as the patient feels the grief to be at a more manageable level.

Imaginal Conversation

The final PGDT procedure is introduced in the closing sequence. This is the *imaginal conversation* with the deceased, which is the main procedure to foster a sense of ongoing connection with the person who died. This is usually done in Session 11, but there is flexibility in the timing, based on when the patient completes the imaginal revisiting sequence. The procedure for an imaginal conversation is to ask the patient to close her eyes and envision herself with the deceased loved one shortly after the death. The patient is asked to imagine that the deceased person can hear and respond. The patient talks to her loved one out loud, asking them or telling them anything the patient wishes. The patient then takes the role of the deceased person and answers, also out loud. Most people have some trepidation in doing this, but once they do, they find it a very powerful exercise. Some find it a great comfort to be able to say and hear things never expressed or acknowledged before.

Casey's Imaginal Conversation

Casey is skeptical about doing the imaginary conversation but agrees to try with the therapist's encouragement. Although her grief is undoubtedly in a different place from when she started the therapy, she still has some worrisome thoughts—for example, that she failed as a mother. The therapist encourages her to use the imaginal conversation to ask those remaining questions. Once ready, Casey closes her eyes, pauses for a while, and says, "Daniel, I love you. I miss you so much every day. I am so sorry I could not protect you and you died alone. I should have been a better mother to you. I feel so guilty for not taking better care of you!" Then she pauses again, her voice changes, and she replies, taking Daniel's role. "I am also sorry, Mom. I wish things had turned out differently, but it is over now. I am not struggling, not suffering anymore. And I want you to know that you were a great mom to me. You were always on my side. Remember, I even wrote it to you in a letter? I love you, mom. Don't worry, I always knew you loved me and wanted the best for me." When Casey stops and opens her eyes, she shares that she is surprised by how comforting this imaginal conversation turned out to be, by the sense of connection to her son she felt. She also comments that she forgot about the letters he wrote when he was sober, expressing his appreciation to her. Remembering those letters was a powerful antidote to her self-doubt and guilt.

Each of the closing sequence sessions addresses treatment termination. The therapist and patient reflect on the treatment together, highlighting progress and identifying activities the patient might want to continue. The therapist helps the patient identify her ongoing strengths and see where vulnerabilities might lie as she thinks about plans for the future. They discuss potentially difficult times ahead and how the patient might handle them. They talk about thoughts and feelings about ending treatment. The time allotted for termination discussions increases gradually from Session 11 to Session 15. The termination discussion culminates in Session 16, reviewing the PGDT model, personalizing the discussion, and highlighting achievements and continuing goals.

Casey's Last Session

At the end of the treatment, Casey's grief feels very different from when she started. She still feels sad when she thinks of Daniel and occasionally has a wave of intense longing, but those waves do not stop her in her tracks and do not take over her day anymore. She no longer holds herself responsible for Daniel's death. She comments with a chuckle that she now has some exciting things to look forward to and doesn't want to kill herself. She is able to better concentrate on her work and feels more satisfied with it. Casey now feels free to leave her house, to see friends, and proudly tells the therapist that she has not declined a social invitation. She also really enjoys her photography class and spends hours on her newfound hobby. "I am so glad I found you and tried this treatment!" exclaims Casey as she gives the therapist a goodbye hug. "I am so grateful to have my life back!"

A Brief Overview of the Development and Testing of PGDT

Major Clinical Trials of PGDT

PGDT was developed in the late 1990s, shortly after publication of the Inventory of Complicated Grief (ICG) (Prigerson et al. 1995), which established thresholds and was a valid, reliable way of identifying an individual with this condition even before there were formal diagnostic criteria in DSM or ICD. Table 7–1 contains a summary of papers reporting treatment outcomes for PGDT. The first pilot study included 21 participants (Shear et al. 2001) ≥3 months after their loss who scored ≥25 on the 19-item ICG. Results showed marked reduction in posttreatment mean ICG score, at less than half the baseline mean. This reduction was nearly twice that previously observed for interpersonal therapy (IPT) in a study targeting bereavement-related depression. Next, with funding from NIMH, we conducted an RCT of PGDT (Shear et al. 2005) in which 95 participants were randomly assigned to receive ~16 sessions of IPT or PGDT. Patients taking psychotropic medication were permitted to enroll. Intent-to-treat analyses of outcome showed a statistically and clinically significant difference between the treatments, with the response rate among PGDT completers being nearly twice that of IPT completers. A secondary analysis of antidepressant medication use showed some differences in both IPT and CGT completion and response rates among those taking concurrent antidepressants. Those results are discussed in more detail in the section Pharmacotherapy.

A second NIMH-funded RCT (Shear et al. 2014) was then conducted for older adults (mean age 66). This trial took place in a different laboratory with different therapists and a population on average more than a decade older than in the first study. Participants scored ≥30 on the ICG and were confirmed in a clinical interview to have grief as their primary problem. Those with a history of psychotic disorder, current substance use, or bipolar I disorder; active suicidality requiring hospitalization; a Mini-Mental Status

Table 7–1. PGD treatment studies

Study	Description
First RCT of PGDT (Shear et al. 2005)	*Active treatment*: 16 sessions of individual therapy over 16–20 weeks
	Study design: Two-arm RCT: PGDT vs. IPT
	Study participants: 102 bereaved adults ≥6 months (median 2.3 years) after loss; ICG ≥30; 87% female; 76% white; age 49±14 years
	Supporting evidence: Response rate greater for PGDT (51%) than IPT (28%); time to response faster for PGDT; NNT 4.3
Analysis of African American study participants in 2005 RCT (Cruz et al. 2007)	*Study design*: Secondary analyses of Shear et al. 2005; contrasted presentation, treatment alliance, and treatment completion/response in two racial groups
	Study participants: 19 African Americans with PGD and 19 white Americans matched for sex, age, and baseline grief severity
	Supporting evidence: No differences were found between the racial groups in any clinical or treatment-related measure
Mediation study of 2005 RCT (Glickman et al. 2017)	*Study design*: Secondary analyses of Shear et al. 2005; examined the mechanisms of action of PGDT
	Study participants: Treatment completers, 35 PGDT and 34 IPT
	Supporting evidence: Reducing avoidance of situations and emotions connected to the loss seems to be a key mechanism of change in PGDT; revising counter-factual thinking around troubling aspects of the death may also play a role in facilitating effective adaptation to loss
RCT of PGDT in older adults (Shear et al. 2014)	*Active treatment*: 16 sessions of individual therapy over 16–20 weeks
	Study design: Two-arm RCT: PGDT vs. IPT
	Study participants: 151 bereaved adults ≥50 years old (66±9); ≥6 months (median 3 years) after loss; ICG ≥30; 82% female; 86% white
	Supporting evidence: Both treatments produced improvement in prolonged grief symptoms (ICG); response rate for PGDT (70.5%) more than twice that for IPT (32.0%); NNT 2.56

Table 7–1.   PGD treatment studies *(continued)*

Study	Description
Mediation study of 2014 RCT (Lechner-Meichsner et al. 2022)	*Study design*: Examined changes in avoidance and maladaptive cognitions as potential mediators of PGDT outcomes using data from Shear et al. 2014
	Study participants: 131 assessment completers
	Supporting evidence: From baseline to week 16, reductions in avoidance mediated reductions in grief symptoms and grief-related impairment, reductions in maladaptive grief-related cognitions mediated treatment response, reductions in grief symptoms, and grief-related impairment; no significant treatment-mediator interactions; could not establish that mediators changed before outcomes; results consistent with theoretical models of PGD and PGDT
RCT of PGDT and antidepressant medication (Shear, Reynolds, Simon, Zisook 2016)	*Active treatment*: PGDT arm, 16 sessions of individual therapy over 16–20 weeks; medication-only arms, 12 weeks of active medication (CIT) or placebo with supportive management
	Study design: Four-arm RCT: PGDT + placebo; PGDT + CIT; placebo; and CIT; conducted at research clinics in New York, Boston, Pittsburgh, and San Diego
	Study participants: 395 bereaved adults ≥ 6 months (mean 7 years) after loss; ICG ≥ 30; 78% female; 82% white; age 53 ± 15 years
	Supporting evidence: PGDT is treatment of choice for PGD; response to PGDT + placebo vs. placebo (82.5% vs. 54.8%; NNT 3.6); CIT did not significantly improve PGDT outcome (PGDT + CIT 83.7% vs. PGDT + placebo 82.5%; NNT 84); only depressive symptoms decreased significantly more when CIT was added to PGDT; by contrast, adding PGDT improved CIT outcome (CIT 69.3% vs. PGDT + CIT 83.7%; NNT 6.9); response to CIT was not significantly different from placebo at week 12 or 20; rates of suicidal ideation diminished to greater extent among participants receiving PGDT vs. those who did not
Study of PTSD in 2016 study (Na et al. 2021)	*Study design*: Examined the presence and response to treatment of PTSSs in bereaved adults with primary PGD using data from Shear, Reynolds, Simon, Zisook 2016

Table 7–1.   PGD treatment studies *(continued)*

Study	Description
	Study participants: all 395 original study participants
	Supporting evidence: Bereavement-related PTSSs are common in bereaved adults with PGD in the context of both violent and nonviolent loss and are associated with poorer functioning; PGDT shows efficacy for PTSSs; CIT does not
Study of suicide bereaved participants in 2016 study (Zisook et al. 2018)	*Study design*: Secondary analyses of Shear, Reynolds, Simon, Zisook 2016 to examine acceptability and effectiveness of antidepressant medication and PGDT for suicide loss survivors
	Study participants: 58 bereaved by suicide, 74 by accident/homicide, and 263 by natural causes
	Supporting evidence: PGDT is an acceptable and promising treatment for suicide bereaved with PGD; medication alone appeared to have low acceptability
Study of African American participants in 2014 and 2016 studies (M. Gacheru, C. Mauro, N. Skritskaya, unpublished observations, 2021)	*Study design*: Secondary analyses of Shear et al. 2014, 2016; compared differences in prolonged grief symptoms and treatment outcomes in participants who self-identified as Black vs. white
	Study participants: 55 Black and 455 white participants with PGD from two clinical trials that examined the efficacy of PGDT
	Supporting evidence: Response rates to PGDT were similar between groups (Blacks 86% vs. whites 78%)
Pilot studies of PGDT	
Shear et al. 2001	*Active treatment*: 16 individual sessions of PGDT over 4 months
	Study design: Pilot open trial of PGDT
	Study participants: 21 bereaved adults ≥3 months (mean 3 years) after loss; ICG ≥25; age 51±16
	Supporting evidence: Significant improvement in grief symptoms (ICG), anxiety (BAI), and depression (BDI) in both ITT and completers
Zuckoff et al. 2006	*Active treatment*: 16 sessions of PGDT front-loaded with eight sessions of motivational interviewing, emotion regulation, and social skills; individual therapy format

Table 7–1.   PGD treatment studies *(continued)*

Study	Description
	Study design: Pilot open trial of PGDT for PGD and comorbid substance use
	Study participants: 16 bereaved adults (9F, 7M); age 42 ± 10 years; mean 10 years since loss; 50% African Americans; 8 completers
	Supporting evidence: Significant reductions in ICG and BDI scores, with large effect sizes
Asukai et al. 2011	*Active treatment*: 12–16 weekly individual 90-minute sessions of Traumatic Grief Treatment Program, a modification of PGDT for traumatic loss with emphasis on in vivo and imaginal exposure while omitting some restoration-oriented components
	Study design: Pilot open trial of treatment for bereaved by violent death
	Study participants: 15 Japanese women with PTSD due to traumatic grief
	Supporting evidence: 13 of 15 participants completed the treatment program; significant reduction in prolonged grief, depression, and PTSD symptom severity at end of treatment and 12-month follow-up
Supiano and Luptak 2014	*Active treatment*: PGDT administered as group therapy, 120-minute sessions over 16 weeks
	Study design: 2-by-4 prospective, randomized controlled clinical trial comparing group PGDT vs. standard group therapy
	Study participants: 39 adults age ≥ 60 years with PGD
	Supporting evidence: Group PGDT participants demonstrated higher treatment response and significantly greater improvement than standard group therapy participants
Nam 2016	*Active treatment*: Modified PGDT, 8 weekly 2-hour sessions
	Study design: RCT comparing PGDT and supportive counseling
	Study participants: 89 South Korean older adults bereaved ≥ 6 months earlier

Table 7–1. **PGD treatment studies** *(continued)*

Study	Description
	Supporting evidence: PGDT produced significantly greater improvement in grief symptoms than supportive counseling; among participants receiving PGDT, those with a supportive person involved in their sessions showed more beneficial results in PGD and depressive symptoms than those without

Note. BAI = Beck Anxiety Inventory; BDI = Beck Depression Inventory; CIT = citalopram; ICG = Inventory of Complicated Grief; IPT = interpersonal therapy; ITT = intention to treat; NNT = number needed to treat; PGD = prolonged grief disorder; PGDT = prolonged grief disorder treatment; PTSS = posttraumatic stress symptom; RCT = randomized controlled trial.

Exam score < 24; a pending lawsuit or disability claim related to the death; or concurrent psychotherapy were excluded. In this study, 151 older adults were randomly assigned to receive 16 sessions of IPT or PGDT. Completion rates were high for both treatments. Intent-to-treat results showed a large difference between PGDT (70.5% responders) and IPT (32.0% responders). Participants taking psychotropic medications were permitted to enroll; moderator analyses, discussed in more detail in the section "Pharmacotherapy," showed no effect on study outcomes.

A third NIMH-funded study included 395 bereaved adults with PGD and was conducted at four sites (New York, Boston, Pittsburgh, and San Diego) to evaluate directly the efficacy of antidepressant medication when administered alone or with PGDT (Shear, Reynolds, Simon, Zisook 2016). Again, participants scored ≥ 30 on the ICG and were confirmed in a clinical interview to have PGD. Those with a history of psychotic disorder or bipolar I disorder, current substance use, active suicidality requiring hospitalization, cognitive impairment, a pending lawsuit or disability claim related to the death, and concurrent psychotherapy or antidepressant treatment were excluded. Results showed a response rate of 83% for PGDT administered with placebo, 55% for placebo without PGDT, 84% for PGDT with citalopram, and 70% for citalopram without PGDT. All pharmacotherapists administered citalopram or placebo with PGDT-informed clinical management; differences in response rates for citalopram or placebo without PGDT were not significant. Medication results of the study are discussed further in the section "Pharmacotherapy."

Other Clinical Trials of PGDT

A pilot study of 16 individuals who met criteria for substance use disorder (seven alcohol, four cannabis, three cocaine, and three methadone) used a 24-session form of PGDT that added eight sessions focused on motivational interviewing, emotion coping, and communication skills to address the substance abuse before starting grief treatment (Zuckoff et al. 2006). Outcome analyses showed a large mean reduction in ICG scores among both completers ($n=8$) and the intent-to-treat group. Percentage of days abstinent also increased significantly for both groups, with medium to large effect sizes before versus after treatment.

Supiano and Luptak (2014) adapted PGDT to use in a group format for older adults. They conducted a pilot study comparing a 16-session group PGDT to a 16-session treatment as usual (TAU) modified from an 8-week grief support group. They randomized two cohorts to each condition: Cohort 1, PGDT $n=11$ and TAU $n=11$; Cohort 2, PGDT $n=9$ and TAU $n=8$. Results showed clinically and statistically significant superiority of group PGDT on response rates and other PGD measures. Additionally, investigators in Japan have studied the effectiveness of PGDT (e.g., S. Nakajima, M. Ito, personal communication, March 2011). In a pilot study of 15 Japanese women who experienced a violent loss, a 12- to 16-session course of modified PGDT produced significant reduction of symptoms from before to after treatment that was maintained through 12 months of follow-up (Asukai et al. 2011).

Additional Treatment Approaches

Cognitive-behavioral Therapy

The basic approach used in PGDT has also been used in several studies of individual (e.g., Boelen et al. 2007; Rosner et al. 2015) and group (e.g., Bryant et al. 2014) cognitive behavioral therapy (CBT). A summary of these studies is provided in Table 7–2 and in Shear (2015).

CBT adapted for prolonged grief has also been shown to be effective in reducing symptoms of PGD. PGDT is an integrative therapy that incorporates modified versions of proven CBT strategies and techniques for PTSD. There are strong similarities between CBT and PGDT, including psychoeducation, symptom monitoring, imaginal and in vivo exposure, some cognitive work, approaches to managing emotional pain or distress related to the death, and working with memories of the deceased. CBT approaches also help patients learn to reengage in life without the deceased; several use be-

Table 7–2. Approaches to Treatment of PGD With RCTs

Study	Treatment
CBT	
Boelen et al. 2007, 2011	*Active treatment*: 12 weekly sessions of exposure therapy plus cognitive restructuring
	In *exposure therapy*, participants tell the story of the loss and identify aspects that are particularly distressing, list internal (thoughts, memories) and external (people, places) items the person avoids, and develop an in vivo exposure plan
	Cognitive restructuring aims to identify, challenge, and change negative cognitions
	Supporting evidence: A multisite study with a total of 54 PGD participants comparing three groups: 1, exposure + cognitive restructuring, 2, cognitive restructuring + exposure, and 3) supportive counseling
Rosner et al. 2014, 2015	*Active treatment*: 20 standard and 5 optional weekly sessions of PG-CBT, mostly 50 minutes, except two 90 minutes; treatment duration 5–11 months
	PG-CBT had three parts: 1) seven sessions on stabilizing and motivating the patient, psychoeducation on normal and prolonged grief and treatment, exploring patient's grief, examination of social roles, daily routines, and their changes; 2) nine sessions, first teaching relaxation, then confrontation and reinterpretation of cognitions and perceptions related to patient, deceased loved ones, and death circumstances; and 3) four sessions, focusing on future prospects and maintaining healthy bond to the deceased
	Treatment uses multiple worksheets and borrows techniques from other therapeutic models such as relaxation techniques, Gestalt therapy, solution-focused brief therapy, multigenerational family therapy, and imagery work; optional sessions are directed toward special situations or occasions such as anniversaries, holidays, birthdays, family sessions, or legal proceedings
	Supporting evidence: A study with 51 PGD participants comparing two treatment arms: PG-CBT and waitlist control (4 months)
Bryant et al. 2014, 2017	*Active treatment*: Ten 2-hour group CBT sessions + four individual exposure sessions

Table 7–2.   Approaches to Treatment of PGD With RCTs *(continued)*

Study	Treatment
	Group CBT includes psychoeducation about grief and PGD, cognitive restructuring of maladaptive appraisals, letter writing to express unresolved issues, facilitating positive memories, discussing goals and relapse prevention at high-risk times
	After Session 2, participants were randomly assigned to receive either exposure therapy (four individual sessions to "relive" for 40 minutes the experience of the death, with distress ratings and therapist focusing them on the most distressing moments; assigned to repeat exposure at least once at home between sessions) or four individual sessions of supportive counseling
	Supporting evidence: A study with 80 PGD participants comparing two treatment arms: 1) group CBT + individual exposure therapy and 2) group CBT + individual supportive counseling
Acierno et al. 2021	*Active treatment*: Seven sessions of weekly BATE-G
	In *BATE-G*, participants generate a list of 10–20 highly defined reinforcing or functional activities in which they can engage to support their personal values and also a list of grief-related avoided activities; these lists are used to plan and do activities
	Supporting evidence: A study with 155 PGD participants comparing two treatment arms: BATE-G and cognitive therapy for grief
Internet-based CBT	
Wagner et al. 2006; Wagner and Maercker 2007 (based on Lange et al. 2000)	*Active treatment*: 5 weeks of CBT for complicated grief consists of two 45-minute writing assignments per week with asynchronous email feedback and instructions from therapist
	CBT protocol is three modules: 1) two essays on circumstances of the death and two on most intrusive moment; 2) two letters to hypothetical friend in similar situation and two focused on rituals to foster new perspectives and new role and identity, to identify lessons learned from the death, and to regain sense of control over lives; 3) two essays to outline important memories regarding the death, reflect on therapeutic process and how the loss has changed them, and describe coping going forward
	Supporting evidence: A study with 55 PGD participants comparing two treatment arms: treatment vs. waiting list

Table 7–2. Approaches to Treatment of PGD With RCTs *(continued)*

Study	Treatment
Kersting et al. 2011 (adaptation of Wagner et al. 2005; 2006 protocol)	*Active treatment*: Internet-based, manualized cognitive behavioral treatment program for complicated grief consisting of 10 writing assignments at scheduled regular intervals
	CBT for mothers after loss of a child during pregnancy consisted of three phases of writing assignments: 1) self-confrontation, four assignments describing the traumatic loss and its circumstances; 2) cognitive restructuring, four assignments, framed as a supportive letter to a hypothetical friend, with the aim of providing new perspectives on the loss; 3) social sharing, two assignments focused on a symbolic farewell letter addressed to themselves, to a person connected with the loss, or to a loved one; twice in each phase, the therapist provided—within one working day—individual written feedback along with instructions on the next writing assignment
	Supporting evidence: A study with 83 PGD participants comparing two treatment arms: treatment vs. waiting list
Eisma et al. 2015	*Active treatment*: Internet-based exposure or behavioral activation: six manual-based emailed homework assignments, completed over 6–8 weeks with therapist written feedback
	Exposure therapy aims to reduce grief-related avoidance by gradual exposure to the most aversive aspects of the loss using a combination of writing assignments and imaginal or in vivo exposure exercises
	Behavioral activation aims to increase meaningful and fulfilling activities that individuals undertake by using an activity diary
	Supporting evidence: A study with 47 PGD participants comparing three treatment arms: exposure, behavioral activation, and waiting list
Treml et al. 2021 (adaptation of Kersting et al. 2011 protocol)	*Active treatment*: Internet-based CBT for complicated grief, 10 writing assignments with therapist feedback over 5 weeks
	CBT for people bereaved by suicide includes 10 writing assignments administered in three phases: self-confrontation, cognitive restructuring, and social sharing
	Supporting evidence: A study with 58 PGD participants comparing two treatment arms: treatment vs. waiting list

**Table 7–2.   Approaches to Treatment of PGD
              With RCTs *(continued)***

Study	Treatment
Kaiser et al. 2022 (adaptation of Kersting et al. 2011 protocol)	*Active treatment*: Internet-based CBT for complicated grief consisting of 10 writing assignments with therapist feedback over 5 weeks CBT for cancer bereavement includes 10 writing assignments administered in three phases: self-confrontation, cognitive restructuring, and social sharing *Supporting evidence*: A study with 87 PGD participants comparing two treatment arms: treatment vs. waiting list
EMDR and ART	
Van Denderen et al. 2018	*Active treatment*: Eight individual sessions of CBT and EMDR for homicidally bereaved *EMDR* + CBT aim to reduce self-rated PGD and PTSD symptoms with two introductory sessions of psychoeducation about homicidal loss and discussion of grief and social support in a joint session with a family member, followed by three 45- to 90-minute sessions of EMDR and three 45-minute sessions of CBT (or vice versa); participants in the immediate condition started the treatment right away, those in the waitlist condition started treatment 4 months later *Supporting evidence*: A study with 85 homicide-bereaved participants with PGD comparing four treatment arms: 1) immediate condition EMDR then CBT; 2) immediate condition CBT then EMDR; 3) waitlist condition EMDR then CBT; 4) waitlist condition CBT then EMDR
Buck et al. 2020	*Active treatment*: Up to 4 weekly 60- to 120-min individual sessions of ART *ART* is brief, protocol-driven, exposure/imagery rescripting therapy that uses lateral left-right eye movements while engaging in a grief-focused activity (e.g., re-experiencing the grief experience and performing eye movements); each session moves though stages of exposure/recall, reduction or elimination of somatic-based distress, and rescripting/resolution to visualize a more positive future *Supporting evidence*: A study with 54 PGD participants comparing two treatment arms: treatment vs. waiting list

Table 7–2. Approaches to Treatment of PGD With RCTs *(continued)*

Study	Treatment
Narrative therapy	
Barbosa et al. 2014 (based on Goncalves 2002)	*Active treatment*: Four weekly 60-minute sessions of cognitive narrative intervention *Cognitive narrative psychotherapy* is manualized brief therapy: session 1 involves recalling narratives to evoke the most difficult episode of loss and to clarify the meaning of the deceased; session 2 involves describing the episode and structuring the experience with sense of authorship, coherence, and diversity of cognitive and emotional content; session 3 involves exploring different meanings of the episode and choosing a metaphor for it; session 4 involves experimenting with the narrative to represent a more adaptive functioning *Supporting evidence*: A study with 40 PGD participants comparing cognitive narrative therapy to a waitlist control

Note. ART=accelerated resolution therapy; BATE-G=behavioral activation and therapeutic exposure for grief; CBT=cognitive behavioral therapy; EMDR=eye movement desensitization and reprocessing; PG-CBT=prolonged grief/cognitive behavioral therapy; PGD=prolonged grief disorder; PGDT=prolonged grief disorder treatment; RCT=randomized controlled trial.

havioral activation approaches. One small pilot study used a strategy focused primarily on encouraging individuals to engage in healthy behaviors and activities to enhance quality of life and reduce negative emotions (Papa et al. 2013).

As elegantly demonstrated by Bryant et al. (2014), however, repeatedly telling the story of the death appears to be a core component of the treatment. Exposure therapy in CBT, as in PGDT, focuses on decreasing avoidance of memories related to the individual's experiences of the death as well as avoidance of painful reminders and situations that remind them of their loved one. Repeatedly confronting these reminders helps the individual feel less distressed by the memories over time (Bryant et al. 2017). This treatment was provided in a group format and used the same approach previously reported for PGDT.

Cognitive restructuring is used formally in CBT for PGD (Boelen et al. 2007; Bryant et al. 2017; Rosner et al. 2014). Cognitive restructuring is a structured, focused way of identifying and modifying thoughts that contribute to painful emotions, as they are generally considered to be unhealthy or maladaptive (Boelen et al. 2007). Virtually all psychotherapy approaches seek to help patients change some of the ways they are thinking, but not all use specific CBT techniques. It is not clear that the way cognitions change is what is relevant. Additionally, a small early study showed that CBT is more effective than supportive counseling only when exposure therapy is administered before cognitive therapy (Boelen et al. 2007).

A range of different CBT protocols have been studied using individual, group, and internet-based formats (e.g., Wagner et al. 2006; Rosner et al. 2014; Eisma et al. 2015; Bryant et al. 2017; see Table 7–2). It is likely that a CBT therapist could provide a good treatment for PGD by ensuring inclusion of the basic elements of PGDT, also used by Bryant et al. (2014) in a group format. Taken together, these studies—along with those of PGDT—strongly suggest that PGD can be treated with short-term therapy, using either a highly structured CBT approach or a more integrated PGDT approach, personalized for both the therapist and the patient.

Alternative Treatment Strategies

Proposals for alternative treatments continue to appear in the literature and to demonstrate promise in improving symptoms of PGD. Table 7–3 includes a summary of these studies. Most publications include just one small study, a clinical case report, or clinical samples. We include them to offer additional resources for clinicians to learn to treat PGD. In addition, it may be that an individual does not yet meet criteria for prolonged grief but is experiencing significant acute grief and seeks support early in the grieving process. In such cases, supportive group or individual interventions should be considered that continue to encourage engagement with grief (rather than avoidance) and engagement in their lives. See Part I, Chapter 4—Clinical Management of a Bereaved Patient by Drs. Zisook and Iglewicz, which discusses various strategies to use when working with a newly grieving person, including empathic listening, normalization, symptom monitoring, and encouragement to engage in life in a meaningful way.

Pharmacotherapy

There is limited evidence from randomized controlled trials supporting pharmacotherapy as an effective treatment in reducing symptoms of PGD, and data available to date support grief-focused psychotherapies as first-line treatment for PGD, based on greater efficacy (Shear, Reynolds, Simon, Zisook 2016). However, antidepressants are commonly used in clinical practice and

Table 7–3. Strategies with Pilot, Open, or Case Studies

Study	Treatment
Cognitive-behavioral approaches	
Papa et al. 2013 (based on Martell et al. 2001 protocol)	*Active treatment*: 12–16 sessions of behavioral activation over 12 weeks
	Behavioral activation treatment includes five stages: 1) session 1, review of assessments, psychoeducation, and defining treatment goals; 2) sessions 2 and 3, introduction of self-monitoring via activities records and practice using them; 3) sessions 4–6, functional assessment to identify links between symptoms and behavior (especially rumination/yearning and other avoidant behavior) and maintaining contingencies, addressing one specific target for activation; 4) sessions 6–10, rehearsal of identifying maladaptive, self-sustaining "grief loops" and implementing alternative behavioral responses while expanding the activation focus to an increasing range of functional problems, including activation homework; 5) session 10 to termination, review of identified grief loops, effective alternative responses, how problems in the implementation of alternative responses were overcome, and how to recognize signs of relapse and respond using activation skills
	Supporting evidence: A pilot study with 25 PGD participants comparing behavioral activation to waiting list
Wenn et al. 2019	*Active treatment*: 6 weekly 2-hour sessions of group metacognitive grief therapy
	Metacognitive grief therapy focuses on modifying unhelpful thought processes such as rumination and worry; it uses various therapeutic techniques, such as detached mindfulness, attention training technique, and behavioral experiments
	Supporting evidence: A study with 22 PGD participants comparing two treatment arms: treatment vs. waiting list
Karangoda et al. 2021	6 weekly sessions of adapted *BATD-R*
	Supporting evidence: 2 PGD cases
Combined therapy	
de Heus et al. 2017	*Active treatment*: 16-session day patient treatment program for refugees

Table 7–3.   Strategies with Pilot, Open, or Case Studies *(continued)*

Study	Treatment
	BEP-TG for refugees embeds individual traumatic grief-focused therapy in group-based multidisciplinary day patient treatment, comprising a weekly 5-hour program consisting of three phases, duration 4 months each
	Supporting evidence: Open treatment of 16 PGD participants
Ohye et al. 2022	*Active treatment*: 2-week intensive outpatient treatment (>61 hours)
	Intensive outpatient program for widows bereaved by the suicide of veteran spouse, with integrative health approaches, combination of evidence-based individual and group psychotherapies targeting PTSD and complicated grief, and skills for stress management, emotion regulation, distress tolerance
	Supporting evidence: Open treatment of 24 participants with both PGD and PTSD
Narrative therapy	
Elinger et al. 2021 (partly based on Peri et al. 2016)	*Active treatment*: 16 weekly 60-minute weekly sessions of narrative reconstruction therapy
	Narrative reconstruction is time-limited integrative therapy consisting of 1) exposure to loss memory through retelling; 2) systematic detailed written reconstruction of loss memory narrative; 3) integration of traumatic memory with other autobiographical memories; and 4) elaboration of the personal significance and subjective meaning of that memory for the bereaved
	Supporting evidence: Open treatment, 16 PGD participants
Lichtenthal et al. 2019	*Active treatment*: 16 weekly 60- to 90-minute sessions, in person or through video, of meaning-centered grief therapy for parents who lost a child to cancer
	Meaning-centered grief therapy is one-on-one cognitive-behavioral/existential intervention using psychoeducation, experiential exercises, and structured discussion to explore meaning, identity, purpose, and legacy
	Supporting evidence: Open treatment of eight PGD participants

Table 7–3. Strategies with Pilot, Open, or Case Studies *(continued)*

Study	Treatment
Vogel et al. 2021	*Active treatment*: 20–24 sessions of PCT, 50 minutes each
	PCT manual for PTSD adapted for use with PGD patients includes education on grief symptoms and daily monitoring of stressors and problems related to PGD and on their active mastery
	Supporting evidence: Open treatment of 20 PGD participants
Music therapy	
Iliya 2015	*Active treatment*: Music therapy in addition to usual care
	In grief-specific music therapy participants sing improvised imaginal dialogues with their deceased loved ones
	Supporting evidence: A study of 10 PGD participants comparing two treatment arms: music therapy with usual care vs. usual care only

Note. BATD-R=behavioral activation for depression, revised; BEP-TG=brief eclectic psychotherapy for traumatic grief; PCT=present-centered therapy; PGD=prolonged grief disorder; PGDT=prolonged grief disorder treatment; PTSD=posttraumatic stress disorder.

may be a reasonable approach when grief-focused psychotherapy approaches are not available, particularly when prolonged grief co-occurs with depression or anxiety, and antidepressants may be a useful augmentation approach for co-occurring depression (Shear et al. 2005; 2014; 2016). Some early studies did find support for depression, but not significant changes in grief (bereavement-related depression in a randomized controlled trial with the tricyclic nortriptyline [Reynolds et al. 1999] and open-label studies of tricyclics or bupropion [Jacobs et al. 1987; Pasternak et al. 1991; Zisook et al. 2001]). Small open-label trials (Bui et al. 2012; Simon 2013) were initially suggestive of potential effectiveness of the use of antidepressants, but not benzodiazepines, in treating prolonged grief.

The only fully powered large randomized controlled trial of an antidepressant for those with a primary diagnosis of PGD, the four-arm HEAL trial, compared the SSRI citalopram with a pill placebo, with or without PGDT. The study failed to find efficacy of citalopram for the primary PGD outcomes but did find greater benefit for co-occurring depression in the

PGDT + citalopram group versus PGDT + placebo (Shear, Reynolds, Simon, Zisook 2016). Earlier smaller (and less controlled) studies support this notion that augmentation with antidepressants may be a useful strategy, particularly for co-occurring depression. For example, there was significantly less dropout from PGDT for those on an antidepressant naturalistically (initiated before the study and continued stably) (91% completion) than those not (58% completion) in a study of PGDT versus IPT (Simon et al. 2008).

As we continue to study the neurobiology, psychophysiology, and clinical psychopathology of this newly defined disorder, additional targeted approaches or further refinements of current therapeutic strategies may emerge. One interesting area of current clinical trials research, for example, draws on the observations of reward system dysfunction (O'Connor et al. 2008; Robinaugh et al. 2016; Kakarala et al. 2020) to investigate the potential of naltrexone as a therapeutic agent for PGD (Prigerson 2020; Gang et al. 2021). Additionally, the neuropeptide oxytocin, which has been implicated in attachment functioning as well as reward system activity, has been an early target of study in grief (Bui et al. 2019). Much more research is needed to better understand if more targeted pharmacotherapies may have a role in the treatment of PGD.

In the meanwhile, grief-focused evidence-based psychotherapies are highly efficacious and are the clear first-line approach to this condition, keeping in mind that there may be a role for pharmacotherapy targeting co-occurring depression and other disorders.

References

Acierno R, Kauffman B, Muzzy W, et al: Behavioral activation and therapeutic exposure vs. cognitive therapy for grief among combat veterans: a randomized clinical trial of bereavement interventions. Am J Hosp Palliat Care 38(12):1470–1478, 2021 33504175

American Psychiatric Association: Diagnostic and Statistical Manual of Mental Disorders, 5th Edition. Arlington, VA, American Psychiatric Association, 2013

American Psychiatric Association: Diagnostic and Statistical Manual of Mental Disorders, 5th Edition, Text Revision. Washington, DC, American Psychiatric Association, 2022

Asukai N, Tsuruta N, Saito A: Pilot study on traumatic grief treatment program for Japanese women bereaved by violent death. J Trauma Stress 24(4):470–473, 2011 21780192

Barbosa V, Sá M, Carlos Rocha J: Randomised controlled trial of a cognitive narrative intervention for complicated grief in widowhood. Aging Ment Health 18(3):354–362, 2014 24073815

Boelen PA, Prigerson HG: The influence of symptoms of prolonged grief disorder, depression, and anxiety on quality of life among bereaved adults: a prospective study. European Archives of Psychiatry and Clinical Neuroscience 257(8):444–452, 2007

Boelen PA, de Keijser J, van den Hout MA, et al.: Treatment of complicated grief: a comparison between cognitive-behavioral therapy and supportive counseling. J Consult Clin Psychol 75(2):277–284, 2007

Boelen PA, de Keijser J, van den Hout MA, et al.: Factors associated with outcome of cognitive-behavioural therapy for complicated grief: a preliminary study. Clin Psychol Psychother 18(4):284–291, 2011

Bowlby J: Attachment and Loss: Volume III: Loss, Sadness and Depression. New York, Basic Books, 1980

Bryant RA, Kenny L, Joscelyne A, et al: Treating prolonged grief disorder: a randomized clinical trial. JAMA Psychiatry 71(12):1332–1339, 2014 25338187

Bryant RA, Kenny L, Joscelyne A, et al: Treating prolonged grief disorder: a 2-year follow-up of a randomized controlled trial. J Clin Psychiatry 78(9):1363–1368, 2017 28445631

Buck HG, Cairns P, Emechebe N, et al: Accelerated resolution therapy: randomized controlled trial of a complicated grief intervention. Am J Hosp Palliat Care 37(10):791–799, 2020 31960705

Bui E, Nadal-Vicens M, Simon NM: Pharmacological approaches to the treatment of complicated grief: rationale and a brief review of the literature. Dialogues Clin Neurosci 14(2):149–157, 2012 22754287

Bui E, Hellberg SN, Hoeppner SS, et al: Circulating levels of oxytocin may be elevated in complicated grief: a pilot study. Eur J Psychotraumatol 10(1):1646603, 2019 31489134

Cruz M, Scott J, Houck P, et al: Clinical presentation and treatment outcome of African Americans with complicated grief. Psychiatr Serv 58(5):700–702, 2007 17463353

de Heus A, Hengst SMC, de la Rie SM, et al: Day patient treatment for traumatic grief: preliminary evaluation of a one-year treatment programme for patients with multiple and traumatic losses. Eur J Psychotraumatol 8(1):1375335, 2017 29038679

DeVaul RA, Zisook S: Psychiatry: unresolved grief. Clinical considerations. Postgrad Med 59(5):267–271, 1976 1264920

Eisma MC, Boelen PA, van den Bout J, et al: Internet-based exposure and behavioral activation for complicated grief and rumination: a randomized controlled trial. Behav Ther 46(6):729–748, 2015 26520217

Elinger G, Hasson-Ohayon I, Barkalifa E, et al: Narrative reconstruction therapy for prolonged grief disorder—a pilot study. Eur J Psychotraumatol 12(1):1896126, 2021 33968326

Gang J, Kocsis J, Avery J, et al: Naltrexone treatment for prolonged grief disorder: study protocol for a randomized, triple-blinded, placebo-controlled trial. Trials 22(1):110, 2021 33522931

Glickman K, Shear MK, Wall MM: Mediators of outcome in complicated grief treatment. J Clin Psychol 73(7):817–828, 2017 27755654

Gonçalves K: Psicoterapia Cognitiva Narrativa: Manual de Terapia Breve [Cognitive Narrative Psychotherapy: Handbook of Brief Therapy]. Bilbao, Spain, Editorial Desclée, 2002

Horowitz MJ, Bonanno GA, Holen A: Pathological grief: diagnosis and explanation. Psychosom Med 55(3):260–273, 1993 8346334

Iliya YA: Music therapy as grief therapy for adults with mental illness and complicated grief: a pilot study. Death Stud 39(1–5):173–184, 2015 25730407

Jacobs SC, Nelson JC, Zisook S: Treating depressions of bereavement with antidepressants. A pilot study. Psychiatr Clin North Am 10(3):501–510, 1987 3684751

Kaiser J, Nagl M, Hoffmann R, et al: Therapist-assisted web-based intervention for prolonged grief disorder after cancer bereavement: randomized controlled trial. JMIR Ment Health 9(2):e27642, 2022 35133286

Kakarala SE, Roberts KE, Rogers M, et al: The neurobiological reward system in Prolonged Grief Disorder (PGD): a systematic review. Psychiatry Res Neuroimaging 303:111135, 2020 32629197

Karangoda MD, Breen LJ, Mazzucchelli TG: Brief behavioural activation for prolonged grief disorder: a case series. Clin Psychol 25(1):88–97, 2021

Kersting A, Kroker K, Schlicht S, et al: Efficacy of cognitive behavioral internet-based therapy in parents after the loss of a child during pregnancy: pilot data from a randomized controlled trial. Arch Womens Ment Health 14(6):465–477, 2011 22006106

Lange A, Schrieken B, Van de Ven J-P, et al: "Interapy": the effects of a short protocolled treatment of posttraumatic stress and pathological grief through the internet. Behav Cogn Psychother 28(2):175–192, 2000

Latham AE, Prigerson HG: Suicidality and bereavement: complicated grief as psychiatric disorder presenting greatest risk for suicidality. Suicide Life Threat Behav 34(4):350–362, 2004 15585457

Lechner-Meichsner F, Mauro C, Skritskaya NA, Shear MK: Change in avoidance and negative grief-related cognitions mediates treatment outcome in older adults with prolonged grief disorder. Psychother Res 32(1): 91–103, 2022 33818302

Lichtenthal WG, Catarozoli C, Masterson M, et al: An open trial of meaning-centered grief therapy: rationale and preliminary evaluation. Palliat Support Care 17(1):2–12, 2019 30683164

Martell CR, Addis ME, Jacobson NS: Depression in Context: Strategies for Guided Action. New York, WW Norton and Co., 2001

Mauro C, Tumasian RA III, Skritskaya N, et al: The efficacy of complicated grief therapy for DSM-5-TR prolonged grief disorder. World Psychiatry 21(2):318–319, 2022 35524621

Na PJ, Adhikari S, Szuhany KL, et al: Posttraumatic distress symptoms and their response to treatment in adults with prolonged grief disorder. J Clin Psychiatry 82(3):20m13576, 2021 34000119

Nam I: Complicated grief treatment for older adults: the critical role of a supportive person. Psychiatry Res 244:97–102, 2016 27479098

O'Connor M-F, Wellisch DK, Stanton AL, et al: Craving love? Enduring grief activates brain's reward center. Neuroimage 42(2):969–972, 2008 18559294

Ohye B, Moore C, Charney M, et al: Intensive outpatient treatment of PTSD and complicated grief in suicide-bereaved military widows. Death Stud 46(2):501–507, 2022

Papa A, Sewell MT, Garrison-Diehn C, Rummel C: A randomized open trial assessing the feasibility of behavioral activation for pathological grief responding. Behav Ther 44(4):639–650, 2013 24094789

Pasternak RE, Reynolds CF III, Schlernitzauer M, et al: Acute open-trial nortriptyline therapy of bereavement-related depression in late life. J Clin Psychiatry 52(7):307–310, 1991 2071562

Peri T, Hasson-Ohayon I, Garber S, et al: Narrative reconstruction therapy for prolonged grief disorder—rationale and case study. Eur J Psychotraumatol 7:30687, 2016 27150596

Prigerson HG (PI): Naltrexone Treatment for Prolonged Grief Disorder (PGD). ClinicalTrials.gov NCT04547985, 2020. Available at: https://clinicaltrials.gov/ct2/show/NCT04547985?term=naltrexone&cond=Grief&cntry=US&draw=2&rank=1. Accessed March 20, 2023.

Prigerson HG, Maciejewski PK, Reynolds CF III, et al: Inventory of Complicated Grief: a scale to measure maladaptive symptoms of loss. Psychiatry Res 59(1–2):65–79,1995 8771222

Prigerson HG, Bierhals AJ, Kasl SV, et al: Traumatic grief as a risk factor for mental and physical morbidity. Am J Psychiatry 154(5):616–623, 1997 9137115

Prigerson HG, Horowitz MJ, Jacobs SC, et al: Prolonged grief disorder: psychometric validation of criteria proposed for DSM-V and ICD-11. PLoS Med 6(8):e1000121,2009 19652695

Reynolds CF III, Miller MD, Pasternak RE, et al: Treatment of bereavement-related major depressive episodes in later life: a controlled study of acute and continuation treatment with nortriptyline and interpersonal psychotherapy. Am J Psychiatry 156(2):202–208, 1999 9989555

Robinaugh DJ, Mauro C, Bui E, et al: Yearning and its measurement in complicated grief. J Loss Trauma 21(5):410–420, 2016

Rosner R, Pfoh G, Kotoučová M, Hagl M: Efficacy of an outpatient treatment for prolonged grief disorder: a randomized controlled clinical trial. J Affect Disord 167:56–63, 2014 25082115

Rosner R, Bartl H, Pfoh G, et al: Efficacy of an integrative CBT for prolonged grief disorder: a long-term follow-up. J Affect Disord 183:106–112, 2015 26001670

Shear K: Adapting imaginal exposure to the treatment of complicated grief, in Pathological Anxiety: Emotional Processing in Etiology and Treatment, New York, Guilford Press, 2006

Shear MK: Clinical practice. Complicated grief. N Engl J Med 372(2):153–160, 2015 25564898

Shear MK, Frank E, Foa E, et al: Traumatic grief treatment: a pilot study. Am J Psychiatry 158(9):1506–1508, 2001 11532739

Shear K, Frank E, Houck PR, Reynolds CF III: Treatment of complicated grief: a randomized controlled trial. JAMA 293(21):2601–2608, 2005 15928281

Shear K, Monk T, Houck P, et al: An attachment-based model of complicated grief including the role of avoidance. Eur Arch Psychiatry Clin Neurosci 257(8):453–461, 2007 17629727

Shear MK, Wang Y, Skritskaya N, et al: Treatment of complicated grief in elderly persons: a randomized clinical trial. JAMA Psychiatry 71(11):1287–1295, 2014 25250737

Shear MK, Reynolds CF III, Simon NM, Zisook S, et al. Optimizing treatment of complicated grief: a randomized clinical trial. JAMA Psychiatry 73(7):685–694, 2016 27276373

Simon NM: Treating complicated grief. JAMA 310(4):416–423, 2013 23917292

Simon NM, Shear MK, Fagiolini A, et al: Impact of concurrent naturalistic pharmacotherapy on psychotherapy of complicated grief. Psychiatry Res 159(1–2):31–36, 2008 18336918

Skritskaya NA, Mauro C, Olonoff M, et al: Measuring maladaptive cognitions in complicated grief: introducing the Typical Beliefs Questionnaire. Am J Geriatr Psychiatry 25(5):541–550, 2017 27793576

Stroebe M, Schut H, Finkenauer C: The traumatization of grief? A conceptual framework for understanding the trauma-bereavement interface. Is J Psychiatry Relat Sci 38(3–4):185–201, 2001 11725417

Supiano KP, Luptak M: Complicated grief in older adults: a randomized controlled trial of complicated grief group therapy. Gerontologist 54(5):840–856, 2014 23887932

Treml J, Nagl M, Linde K, et al: Efficacy of an Internet-based cognitive-behavioural grief therapy for people bereaved by suicide: a randomized controlled trial. Eur J Psychotraumatol 12(1):1926650, 2021 34992754

Van Denderen M, de Keijser J, Stewart R, Boelen PA: Treating complicated grief and posttraumatic stress in homicidally bereaved individuals: a randomized controlled trial. Clin Psychol Psychother 2018 29479767

Vogel A, Comtesse H, Nocon A, et al: Feasibility of present-centered therapy for prolonged grief disorder: results of a pilot study. Front Psychiatry 12:534664, 2021 33935813

Wagner B, Maercker A: A 1.5-year follow-up of an Internet-based intervention for complicated grief. J Trauma Stress 20(4):625–629, 2007 17721955

Wagner B, Knaevelsrud C, Maercker A: Internet-based treatment for complicated grief: concepts and case study. J Loss Trauma 10(5):409–432, 2005

Wagner B, Knaevelsrud C, Maercker A: Internet-based cognitive-behavioral therapy for complicated grief: a randomized controlled trial. Death Stud 30(5):429–453, 2006 16610157

Wenn JA, O'Connor M, Kane RT, et al: A pilot randomised controlled trial of metacognitive therapy for prolonged grief. BMJ Open 9(1):e021409, 2019 30782672

Zisook S, Shuchter SR, Pedrelli P, et al: Bupropion sustained release for bereavement: results of an open trial. J Clin Psychiatry 62(4):227–230, 2001 11379835

Zisook S, Shear MK, Reynolds CF, et al: Treatment of complicated grief in survivors of suicide loss: a HEAL report. J Clin Psychiatry 79(2):17m11592, 2018 29617064

Zuckoff A, Shear K, Frank E, et al: Treating complicated grief and substance use disorders: a pilot study. J Subst Abuse Treat 30(3):205–211, 2006 16616164

8

Conclusion

Charles F. Reynolds, III, M.D.
Stephen Cozza, M.D.
Paul Maciejewski, Ph.D.
Holly Prigerson, Ph.D.
M. Katherine Shear, M.D.
Naomi M. Simon, M.D.
Sidney Zisook, M.D.
Natalia Skritskaya, Ph.D.

We know that loss is inevitable in life, that "grief is an innate part of what it means to live a full and rich life as a human." So wrote A.C. Shilton (2021) in "There Is No Vaccine for Grief." In other words, grief follows from love and close attachment to others and thus is inextricably bound with a life filled with meaning, joy, connection, and sorrow.

Shilton's question "Can one fortify oneself for grief?" is foundational for the readers of this handbook—indeed, for all of us, because grief is universal. Can one nourish resilience to navigate the journey of grief and protect oneself from grief being prolonged and disabling? It seems particularly appropriate and timely to address this issue head-on in a handbook whose primary raison d'être is to offer guidance to both clinical and lay readers.

Shilton suggests that it may be possible to prepare oneself for grief and advocates five broad strategies for doing so:

1. "[Practice] experiencing your emotions";
2. "Shower the people you love with love";

3. "Nurture your network";
4. "Recognize your coping style"; and
5. "Find a natural space."

In the foreword to this handbook, we contextualized the clinical management of grief and its complications within a broader framework, including the COVID-19 pandemic. To elaborate: we can inoculate ourselves against the COVID-19 virus and its variants, or more precisely, against its complications: severe illness, long-haul disability, and death. We know that behavioral measures, based in public health, are central to reducing viral spread and replication and, thereby, the genesis of even more transmissible and potentially lethal variants, such as Delta and Omicron.

By analogy, and extending the metaphor, we ask whether there is a "vaccine," as it were, that could inoculate us against prolonged suffering, disability, and suicide—born of the inability of grievers and their supporting friends and family to recognize and set aside early defensive processes that entail turning away from the reality of the loss. Put differently, and more affirmatively, is there a vaccine that could nourish resilience, so that one's "bank account" of resilience is available in the face of losing a loved one? Can such inoculation enable a healthier, more adaptive response and prevent complications such as prolonged grief disorder?

This question is about the science of preventing PGD. But the answer can be informed by strategies that facilitate natural adaptive processes oriented toward accepting reality and restoring the capacity for well-being in the days, weeks, and months after the loss of a loved one.

Drawing on another metaphor: a wound heals naturally in the absence of complications, such as infection or diabetes, that interfere with the body's restorative processes. By analogy, an important loss brings a myriad of disruptive changes that evoke natural adaptive healing responses. As adaptation progresses, the experience of a loss changes, the new reality becomes integrated into ongoing life, and grief follows suit. But the process of adapting can be derailed if a griever's initial defensive coping responses persist and are overly influential in mental functioning (Bowlby 1980)—and perhaps for other reasons that continue to be investigated. When adaptation is stalled, the experience of the loss remains fresh and grievers get stuck in the throes of acute grief, which only reinforces the use of defensive coping. The architecture of risk and protection against PGD, still an evolving science, is becoming clearer.

We are fortunate that there are evidence-based, short-term methods to treat PGD. We look forward to a time when we will also know specific strategies for building resilience, helping those with acute grief to learn how to navigate the journey in an adaptive way, and thereby protecting against the development of PGD.

Prolonged grief disorder therapy (PGDT; previously, complicated grief therapy, CGT), as described by Skritskaya et al. in Chapter 7 of this handbook, involves facilitating the adaptation to loss and addressing impediments to that process. The process of adapting is operationalized as a series of "healing milestones": understanding and accepting grief, managing grief-related emotions (both painful and pleasurable), seeing possibilities for future happiness, strengthening relationships, narrating a story of the death, living with reminders, and feeling a connection to the person who died. Common "derailers" are identified and addressed, in particular those centered on counterfactual thinking and avoidance, both behavioral and experiential.

PGDT is an integrative therapy that is built on a large body of research. Principles and strategies are informed by laboratory research findings from, for example, attachment; caregiving; exploration; other research pertaining to close relationships; self-determination and other studies in positive psychology; cognitive processes; coping and adapting; emotion regulation; experiential avoidance; reward conditioning; and extinction processes. The intervention strategies and techniques are derived from prolonged exposure therapy for PTSD (understanding grief, narrating the story of the death, living with reminders), interpersonal psychotherapy (strengthening relationships, role transition strategies), motivational interviewing (seeing a promising future), emotion-focused therapy (managing grief-related emotional pain), positive psychology (managing grief-related emotions, seeing a positive future, strengthening relationships), and psychodynamic psychotherapy (active listening, self-observation, reflection). The principles and procedures used successfully to redirect adaptation to loss in PGDT can also be applied to help those struggling with acute grief—diagnosable in DSM-5-TR (American Psychiatric Association 2022) as "uncomplicated bereavement."

The key clinical and scientific point, in conclusion, is the need to build and to test hypotheses addressing the prevention of prolonged grief disorder and, equally with respect to both prevention and treatment, to determine what works for whom, how, and when. As our field has learned in depression prevention and treatment research, this type of investigation is vital to bridging intervention science with clinical care. At the same time, progress in understanding the neurobiological substrates of PGD is accelerating through the availability of tools for functional brain imaging and measuring peripheral molecules, such as endocannabinoids, which moderate stress responses (Chen et al. 2020; Kang et al. 2021; Reiland et al. 2021). Brain network biomarkers of emotion dysregulation and dysfunctional reward processing may serve as predictors of worsening grief trajectories, including the development of PGD and accompanying psychiatric complications such as MDD and PTSD.

Moreover, given the availability of a highly effective, specific, and safe treatment—PGDT—we can now ask and seek answers to questions about the moderators and mediators of treatment effectiveness. How does PGDT work, and for whom? When should it be administered? We can use PGDT as a probe to better understand the mechanisms by which depression, PTSD, and loneliness pose risk for complicating and prolonging the course of grief.

The authors hope that this handbook will further stimulate such science and its translation into real-world care. Most of us—if not all of us—will need the fruits of such science sooner or later, as well as the loving care we trust and hope it may beget.

References

American Psychiatric Association: Diagnostic and Statistical Manual of Mental Disorders, 5th Edition, Text Revision. Washington, DC, American Psychiatric Association, 2022

Bowlby J: Disordered variants, in Attachment and Loss, Volume III, Loss, Sadness and Depression, New York: Basics Books, 1980, pp 140

Chen G, Ward BD, Claesges SA, et al: Amygdala functional connectivity features in grief: a pilot longitudinal study. Am J Geriatr Psychiatry 28(10):1089–1101, 2020 32253102

Kang M, Bohorquez-Montoya L, McAuliffe T, et al: Loneliness, circulating endocannabinoid concentrations, and grief trajectories in bereaved older adults: a longitudinal study. Front Psychiatry 12:783187, 2021 34955928

Reiland H, Banerjee A, Claesges SA, et al: The influence of depression on the relationship between loneliness and grief trajectories in bereaved older adults. Psychiatry Res Commun 1(1):100006, 2021 35928209

Shilton AC: There is no vaccine for grief. The New York Times, March 21, 2021, page D6

APPENDIX A

Prolonged Grief Disorder (PG-13-Revised)

Holly G. Prigerson, Ph.D., Jiehui Xu, M.S., Paul K. Maciejewski, Ph.D.

Q1. Have you lost someone significant to you? ◯ Yes   ◯ No

Q2. How many months has it been since your significant other died?   18   months

For each item below, please indicate how you currently feel?

Since the death, or as a result of the death...	Not at all	Slightly	Somewhat	Quite a bit	Overwhelmingly
Q3. Do you feel yourself longing or yearning for the person who died?	◯	◯	◯	◯	◯
Q4. Do you have trouble doing the things you normally do because you are thinking so much about the person who died?	◯	◯	◯	◯	◯
Q5. Do you feel confused about your role in life or feel like you don't know who you are any more (i.e., feeling like that a part of you has died) ?	◯	◯	◯	◯	◯
Q6. Do you have trouble believing that the person who died is really gone?	◯	◯	◯	◯	◯
Q7. Do you avoid reminders that the person who died is really gone?	◯	◯	◯	◯	◯
Q8. Do you feel emotional pain, sorrow, or pangs of grief about the death?	◯	◯	◯	◯	◯
Q9. Do you feel that you have trouble re-engaging in life (e.g., problems engaging with friends, pursuing interests, planning for the future)?	◯	◯	◯	◯	◯
Q10. Do you feel emotionally numb or detached from others?	◯	◯	◯	◯	◯
Q11. Do you feel that life is meaningless without the person who died?	◯	◯	◯	◯	◯
Q12. Do you feel alone or lonely without the deceased?	◯	◯	◯	◯	◯

Q13. Have the symptoms above caused significant impairment in social, occupational, or other important areas of functioning?   ◯ Yes / ◯ No

Your summed score is_____.   Interpret

183

APPENDIX B

Structured Clinical Interview for Prolonged Grief Disorder

Holly G. Prigerson, Ph.D.
Martin Viola, M.A.
Wendy Lichtenthal, Ph.D.
Madeline Rogers, L.C.S.W.
Heather M. Derry, Ph.D.
Wan Jou She, Ph.D.
Janna Gordon-Elliott, M.D.
Paul K. Maciejewski, Ph.D.

Instructions

Standard administration of the Structured Clinical Interview for Prolonged Grief Disorder (SCIP) is needed to ensure reliable and valid scoring and diagnosis. SCIP should be administered by interviewers who have received training in structured clinical interviewing and instruction in how to make a differential diagnosis of mental illness in the context of bereavement. This includes a thorough understanding of the conceptual basis of PGD and its various symptoms and detailed knowledge of the features and conventions of SCIP itself.

Administration

1. Identify an index loss to serve as the basis for symptom inquiry. The index loss must involve the death of a significant other.
2. Read prompts verbatim, one at a time, in the order presented, except:

   a. Use the respondent's own words for labeling the loss.

3. In general, do not suggest responses. If a respondent has difficulty understanding a prompt, it may be necessary to offer a brief example to clarify and illustrate. However, this should be done rarely and only after the respondent has been given ample opportunity to answer spontaneously.
4. Move through the interview as efficiently as possible to minimize respondent burden. Some useful strategies:

   a. Be thoroughly familiar with SCIP so that prompts flow smoothly.
   b. Ask the fewest number of prompts needed to obtain sufficient information to support a valid rating.
   c. Minimize note-taking and write while the respondent is talking to avoid long pauses.
   d. Take charge of the interview. Be respectful but firm in keeping the respondent on task, transitioning between questions, pressing for examples, or pointing out contradictions.

Interviewer Scoring

To align with DSM-5-TR criteria for prolonged grief disorder, SCIP assesses the frequency and intensity of symptoms, as well as the extent of functional impairment due to these symptoms. To receive a positive diagnosis of prolonged grief disorder, the following is required:

Criterion A

The indexed loss must have occurred 12 months before the interview for adults or 6 months before for children and adolescents (reported in item A3).

Criterion B

The respondent must report symptoms of yearning and/or preoccupation about the deceased at a clinically significant degree and frequency. This criterion is met by responses of "quite a bit" or "overwhelmingly" to items B1 or B2, indexing clinical significance, and responses of "nearly every day" or "several times a day" to items B1a or B2a, indexing frequency of symptoms. Positive responses are colored in gray.

Criterion C

At least three of the eight listed symptoms in this criterion must be reported at least at the level of clinical intensity and frequency as in Criterion B. This is satisfied by responses of "quite a bit" or "overwhelmingly" for the severity items and "nearly every day" or "several times a day" for the frequency items for at least three of the same symptoms (i.e., C1 and C1a, C2 and C2a, C3 and C3a). Positive responses are colored in gray.

Criterion D

At least one of the four items must be reported as "moderate" or "severe impact." Positive responses are colored in gray.

Criterion E

The grief reaction must exceed cultural norms for the interviewee, in terms of both duration (item E4) and severity (item E5). These items are rated by the interviewer with substantial input from the interviewee, who is the expert on their own cultural context. Grief reactions may vary widely between cultures; in discussing these items, both cultural competency and cultural humility are needed to ensure proper administration and evaluation.

Criterion F

Based on rater evaluation, the symptoms reported by the interviewee are not better explained by another mental disorder, such as major depressive disorder or PTSD, medical condition, or physiological effects of a substance. SCIP does not assess for presence of these factors. Rather, they must independently be ruled out by the interviewer. An evaluation of "no" in item F1 is required for a diagnosis of prolonged grief disorder.

Global Ratings

Overall validity of responses must be evaluated by the interviewer as "excellent" "good," or "fair." Positive responses are colored in gray.

For each section of SCIP, responses necessary to establish a diagnosis of prolonged grief disorder are colored in gray.

Table 1.   Criterion A: Exposure to loss of a significant other

I'm going to ask you about your grief related to the loss of [name]. I'll ask you to share just a little about your relationship with [name], and then I'll ask you about your emotional response to this loss. In general, I do not need a lot of information—just enough so that I can understand any problems that you may have had. Please let me know if you find yourself becoming upset as we go through the questions so that we can slow down and talk about it. Also, let me know if you have any questions or if you don't understand something. Do you have any questions before we start?

A1. I'd like to begin by asking you to tell me briefly about your relationship with [name]. What was your relationship like? Would you describe it as close?

Note to probe: How close were you? What are some ways you would describe your relationship (e.g., close, complicated, dependent)?

_____

_____

_____

The unscored items below may be used to assess potential prior history of PGD.

Just so I have a little more background, may I ask have you experienced any additional deaths of people close to you in the past, other than [name]?

_____

If yes, when did they occur?

_____

If yes, do you feel that your grief reaction was extremely distressing, persistent, and disabling?

_____

Table 2.   Criterion B: Separation distress: the bereaved person experiences yearning or preoccupation with the loss at least daily and at a clinically significant degree

For the remainder of the interview, as I ask you about different feelings and reactions, grief related to [losses previously mentioned] may come up. Please try to keep feelings and reactions related to the loss of [name] in mind as I ask you about different reactions it may have evoked for you. (If you find that it's hard to disentangle your grief over [other losses], please let me know and I'll make a note of it.) You may have experienced some of these thoughts, feelings, and behaviors before the death of [name], but for this interview we're going to focus just on the past month in the period since the death. For each reaction I ask about, I'll ask if you've experienced it in the past month, and if so, how often and how much it bothered you. These questions are multiple choice, so I will ask the question and then present you with the options.

Note: Apologize to the participant that many of these questions may be repeated from your previous conversation.

B1. Do you feel yourself longing or yearning for [name]?

Not at all ☐	Slightly ☐	Somewhat ☐	Quite a bit ☐	Overwhelmingly ☐

If Item B1 = "Quite a bit" or "Overwhelmingly":
B1a. How frequently have you experienced this?

At least once in the past month ☐	At least once a week ☐	Nearly every day ☐	Several times a day ☐	

B2. Have you felt preoccupied with thoughts or memories of [name]?

Not at all ☐	Slightly ☐	Somewhat ☐	Quite a bit ☐	Overwhelmingly ☐

If Item B2 = "Quite a bit" or "Overwhelmingly":
B2a. How frequently have you experienced this?

At least once in the past month ☐	At least once a week ☐	Nearly every day ☐	Several times a day ☐	

Table 3. Criterion C: Cognitive, emotional, and behavioral symptoms: the bereaved person must have three (or more) of the following symptoms experienced at least daily or to a disabling degree

C1. Since the death, or as a result of the death, do you feel confused about your role in life or feel like you don't know who you are any more (i.e., feeling like a part of you has died)?

Not at all ☐	Slightly ☐	Somewhat ☐	Quite a bit ☐	Overwhelmingly ☐

If Item C1 = "Quite a bit" or "Overwhelmingly":
C1a. How frequently have you experienced this?

At least once in the past month ☐	At least once a week ☐	Nearly every day ☐	Several times a day ☐	

C2. Do you have trouble believing that [name] is really gone?

Not at all ☐	Slightly ☐	Somewhat ☐	Quite a bit ☐	Overwhelmingly ☐

If Item C2 = "Quite a bit" or "Overwhelmingly":
C2a. How frequently have you experienced this?

At least once in the past month ☐	At least once a week ☐	Nearly every day ☐	Several times a day ☐	

C3. Do you avoid reminders that [name] is really gone?

Not at all ☐	Slightly ☐	Somewhat ☐	Quite a bit ☐	Overwhelmingly ☐

Table 3.   Criterion C: Cognitive, emotional, and behavioral symptoms: the bereaved person must have three (or more) of the following symptoms experienced at least daily or to a disabling degree *(continued)*

If Item C3 = "Quite a bit" or "Overwhelmingly":
C3a. How frequently have you experienced this?

At least once in the past month ☐	At least once a week ☐	Nearly every day ☐	Several times a day ☐	Overwhelmingly ☐

C4. Do you feel emotional pain (e.g., anger, bitterness, sorrow) related to the death?

Not at all ☐	Slightly ☐	Somewhat ☐	Quite a bit ☐	Overwhelmingly ☐

If Item C4 = "Quite a bit" or "Overwhelmingly":
C4a. How frequently have you experienced this?

At least once in the past month ☐	At least once a week ☐	Nearly every day ☐	Several times a day ☐	

C5. Since the death, or as a result of the death, do you feel that you have trouble re-engaging in life (e.g., problems engaging with friends, pursuing interests, planning for the future)?

Not at all ☐	Slightly ☐	Somewhat ☐	Quite a bit ☐	Overwhelmingly ☐

If Item C5 = "Quite a bit" or "Overwhelmingly":
C5a. How frequently have you experienced this?

At least once in the past month ☐	At least once a week ☐	Nearly every day ☐	Several times a day ☐	

Table 3. Criterion C: Cognitive, emotional, and behavioral symptoms: the bereaved person must have three (or more) of the following symptoms experienced at least daily or to a disabling degree *(continued)*

C6. Since the death, or as a result of the death, do you feel emotionally numb or detached from others?

Not at all ☐	Slightly ☐	Somewhat ☐	Quite a bit ☐	Overwhelmingly ☐

If Item C6 = "Quite a bit" or "Overwhelmingly":
C6a. How frequently have you experienced this?

At least once in the past month ☐	At least once a week ☐	Nearly every day ☐	Several times a day ☐

C7. Do you feel that life is meaningless without [name]?

Not at all ☐	Slightly ☐	Somewhat ☐	Quite a bit ☐	Overwhelmingly ☐

If Item C7 = "Quite a bit" or "Overwhelmingly":
C7a. How frequently have you experienced this?

At least once in the past month ☐	At least once a week ☐	Nearly every day ☐	Several times a day ☐

C8. Do you feel alone or lonely without [name]?

Not at all ☐	Slightly ☐	Somewhat ☐	Quite a bit ☐	Overwhelmingly ☐

If Item C8 = "Quite a bit" or "Overwhelmingly":
C8a. How frequently have you experienced this?

At least once in the past month ☐	At least once a week ☐	Nearly every day ☐	Several times a day ☐

Table 4. Criterion D: The disturbance causes clinically significant distress or impairment in social, occupational, or other important areas of functioning

The following items are asked as open-ended questions and scored by the interviewer to reflect the most appropriate category.

These questions will be open-ended, so you can respond freely.

Significant distress

D1. Overall, in the past month, to what extent have you felt distressed by your grief symptoms?

Note to probe: "Distress": symptoms are upsetting or bothersome; symptoms cause anxiety, frustration, or anger; respondent wishes symptoms/ feelings would go away or were not present (or is worried they will not improve).

☐ Not at all distressed	☐ Mildly distressed ("slightly" or "a little" upset or bothered about the presence of grief symptoms)	☐ Moderately distressed (more than "slightly" or "a little" upset or bothered by the presence of grief symptoms, but not "quite a bit" or overwhelming distress)	☐ Significantly distressed (quite a bit of upset, bother, anxiety, or frustration about the presence of grief symptoms but not overwhelming or all-consuming)	☐ Severely distressed (overwhelmed or consumed by distress related to the presence of grief symptoms)

Social functioning: *consider impairment in social functioning reported on in earlier items*

D2. Overall, in the past month, has your loss affected your relationships with other people? How so? Would you say you felt socially isolated before the death? *If yes:* Was there a marked change in your feelings of social isolation following the death?

☐ No adverse impact	☐ Mild impact, minimal impairment in social functioning	☐ Moderate impact, distress clearly present and significant but not incapacitating	☐ Marked impact, distress clearly present and significantly impairing	☐ Severe impact, considerable distress, socially incapacitated

Table 4. Criterion D: The disturbance causes clinically significant distress or impairment *(continued)* in social, occupational, or other important areas of functioning *(continued)*

Occupational functioning: *consider reported work history, including number and duration of jobs, as well as the quality of work relationships; if premorbid functioning is unclear, inquire about work experiences before the loss.*

D3. *If unclear:* Are you working now? *If yes:* Overall, in the past month, has your loss affected your work or your ability to work?

☐ No adverse impact	☐ Mild impact, minimal impairment in occupational functioning	☐ Moderate impact, definite impairment but not severe occupational dysfunction	☐ Marked impact, distress clearly present and significantly impairing	☐ Severe impact, marked impairment, unable to work

Other functioning

D4. Overall, in the past month, have you had trouble doing any other things you normally do because of your loss?

☐ No adverse impact	☐ Mild impact, minimal impairment in other important areas of functioning	☐ Moderate impact, definite impairment but not severe dysfunction in other important areas of functioning	☐ Marked impact, distress clearly present and significantly impairing	☐ Severe impact, marked impairment, few if any aspects of functioning still intact in specified areas

Table 5.   Criterion E: Severity and duration of grief exceeds social/cultural/religious norms

Next, I would like to ask you some questions about your culture. I'd like to ask these questions to better understand how the way you've been feeling relates to how people like your friends and family may expect you to feel or behave.

E1. Do you feel connected to any social groups, ethnic groups, or traditions? How would you describe your culture? Are you part of multiple cultures?

_____

_____

E2. How do people in your culture or religion experience grief? Are there any rules or traditions about *how* someone like yourself should grieve? Are there any traditions or rules about *how long* someone like yourself should grieve?

_____

_____

E3. In your opinion, is how you feel and act different than what people in your culture expect for someone who is experiencing grief?

_____

_____

E4. *Based on responses of E1–E3, evaluate whether the interviewee's duration of grief symptoms clearly exceeds the social, cultural, or religious norms for their culture and context.*

Does not exceed norms ❑	Exceeds norms ❑

E5. *Based on responses of E1–E3, evaluate whether the interviewee's severity of grief symptoms clearly exceeds the social, cultural, or religious norms for their culture and context.*

Does not exceed norms ❑	Exceeds norms ❑

Table 6.   Criterion F: Differential diagnosis

F1. Are the symptoms reported by the participant better explained by major depressive disorder, posttraumatic stress disorder, or another mental disorder, or attributable to the physiological effects of a substance (e.g., medication, alcohol) or another medical condition?

Yes ❑	No ❑

Table 7.   Global ratings

Estimate the overall validity of responses. Consider factors such as compliance with the interview; mental status (e.g., problems with concentration, comprehension of items, dissociation), and evidence of efforts to exaggerate or minimize symptoms.

☐ Excellent, no reason to suspect invalid responses	☐ Good, factors present that may adversely affect validity	☐ Fair, factors present that may reduce validity	☐ Poor, factors present that clearly reduce validity	☐ Invalid responses, severely impaired mental status or possible deliberate "faking bad" or "faking good"

Estimate the overall severity of PGD symptoms. Consider degree of subjective distress, degree of functional impairment, observations of behaviors in interview, and judgment regarding reporting style.

☐ No clinically significant symptoms, no distress and no functional impairment	☐ Mild, minimal distress or functional impairment	☐ Moderate, definite distress or functional impairment that is not incapacitating	☐ Marked distress or functional impairment that is clearly present and significantly impairing but not incapacitating	☐ Severe, considerable distress or functional impairment, limited functioning even with effort

Index

Page numbers printed in **boldface** type refer to tables and figures.